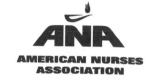

AMERICAN NURSES ASSOCIATION

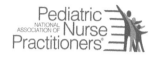

Pediatric
NATIONAL
ASSOCIATION OF Nurse
Practitioners

Society
of
Pediatric
Nurses

Scope and Standards of Practice

Pediatric Nursing

Second Edition

American Nurses Association
Silver Spring, Maryland
2015

The American Nurses Association (ANA), National Association of Pediatric Nurse Practitioners (NAPNAP), and Society of Pediatric Nurses (SPN) are national professional associations. This ANA publication, *Pediatric Nursing: Scope and Standards of Practice, Second Edition*, reflects the thinking of the nursing profession on various issues and should be reviewed in conjunction with state board of nursing policies and practices. State law, rules, and regulations govern the practice of nursing, while *Pediatric Nursing: Scope and Standards of Practice, Second Edition* guides nurses in the application of their professional knowledge, skills, and responsibilities.

American Nurses Association
8515 Georgia Avenue, Suite 400
Silver Spring, MD 20910-3492
1-800-274-4ANA
http://www.Nursingworld.org

Library of Congress Cataloging-in-Publication is on file.

ISBN-13: 978-1-55810-635-2   SAN: 851-3481   02/2016R

First printing: November 2015. Second printing: February 2016.

Contents

Contributors

A work group cochaired by members from the National Association of Pediatric Nurse Practitioners (NAPNAP) and the Society of Pediatric Nurses (SPN), and composed of members of NAPNAP, SPN, the Pediatric Endocrinology Nursing Society (PENS), the Association of Pediatric Gastroenterology and Nutrition Nurses (APGNN), the American Pediatric Surgical Nurses Association (APSNA), and the Society of Pediatric Cardiovascular Nurses (SPCN) developed *Pediatric Nursing: Scope and Standards of Practice, Second Edition* in collaboration with the American Nurses Association. It addresses pediatric nursing practice at all levels and in all settings to assist clinicians, educators, regulators, legislators, and the public.

Scope and Standards Writing Work Group Members

Patricia Clinton, PhD, RN, CPNP, FAANP, FAAN (Cochair, NAPNAP)
University of Iowa, College of Nursing, Iowa City, IA

Wayne Neal, MAT, BSN, RN-BC (Cochair, SPN)
Children's National Medical Health Systems, Washington, DC

Isabel Couto, MSN, RN, CPN, NE-BC (PENS)
Novo Nordisk Inc., Plainsboro, NJ

Cathy Haut, DNP, CPNP-AC, CPNP-PC, CCRN (NAPNAP)
Beacon Pediatrics, Rehoboth Beach, DE; University of Maryland School of Nursing, Baltimore, MD

Jean B. Ivey, PhD, CRNP, PNP-PC, FAANP (NAPNAP and AFPNP)
University of Alabama at Birmingham, Birmingham, AL

Lynette A. Juluke, MSN, RN, CPN (SPN)
Everest College-Tyson's Campus, McLean, VA

Diane Kocovsky, APRN (APGNN)
Boys Town National Research Hospital, Omaha, NE

Mary E. Lynch, RN, MS, MPH, PPCNP-BC, FAAN (SPN)
UCSF School of Nursing, San Francisco, CA

Carmel A. McComiskey, DNP, CRNP, FAANP (APSNA)
University of Maryland Medical Center; University of Maryland School of
Nursing, Baltimore, MD

Mary Rummell, MN, RN, CNS, CPNP, FAHA (SPCN)
Oregon Health & Science University, Portland, OR

Scope and Standards Review Panel Work Group Members

Jan M. Foote, DNP, RN, ARNP, CPNP (PENS)
The University of Iowa College of Nursing, Iowa City, IA; Blank Children's
Hospital, Des Moines, IA

Lisa M. Kohr, RN, MSN, CPNP-AC/PCC, MPH, PhD(c), FCCM (SPCN)
Children's Hospital of Philadelphia, Philadelphia, PA

Lynn Mohr, MS, APN, PCNS-BC, CPN (SPN)
Rush University College of Nursing, Chicago, IL

Lisa Philichi, MN, RN, CPNP (APGNN)
Mary Bridge Children's Hospital and Health Center, Tacoma, WA

Pam Pieper, PhD, ARNP, PNP-BC (APSNA)
University of Florida College of Nursing; University of Florida College of
Medicine, Division of Pediatric Surgery, Jacksonville, FL

Martha K. Swartz, PhD, RN, CPNP, FAAN (NAPNAP)
Yale University School of Nursing, New Haven, CT

ANA Committee on Nursing Practice Standards

Richard Henker, PhD, RN, CRNA, FAAN – Cochair (03/2014–12/2015)

Tresha (Terry) L. Lucas, MSN, RN – Cochair (07/2011–12/2014)

Danette Culver, MSN, APRN, ACNS-BC, CCRN

Deborah Finnell, DNS, PMHNP-BC, CARN-AP, FAAN

Renee Gecsedi, MS, RN

Deedra Harrington, DNP, MSN, APRN, ACNP-BC

Maria Jurlano, MS, BSN, RN, NEA-BC, CCRN

Carla A. B. Lee, PhD, APRN-BC, CNAA, FAAN, FIBA

Verna Sitzer, PhD, RN, CNS

American Nurses Association Staff

Carol J. Bickford, PhD, RN-BC, CPHIMS, FAAN – Content editor

Maureen Cones, JD – Legal counsel

Yvonne Humes, MSA – Project coordinator

Eric Wurzbacher – Project editor

NAPNAP Staff

Dolores C. Jones, EdD, RN, CPNP (Contributor) – Dean, Academic Affairs, Chamberlain College of Nursing

Eileen Arnold – NAPNAP Executive Assistant

About the National Association of Pediatric Nurse Practitioners

The National Association of Pediatric Nurse Practitioners (NAPNAP) is the professional association for pediatric nurse practitioners and other advanced practice registered nurses dedicated to improving the quality of health care for infants, children, adolescents, and young adults. NAPNAP has been advocating for children's health since 1973 and was the first nurse practitioner professional society in the United States. Our mission is to empower nurse practitioners who work in pediatrics and their healthcare partners to enhance child and family health through practice, leadership, advocacy, education, and research. Along with superior clinical expertise and academic knowledge in primary, acute, and specialty health care, NAPNAP members include national child healthcare experts, respected authors, distinguished faculty, and practicing professionals in the delivery of pediatric health care (http://www.napnap.org/).

About the Society of Pediatric Nurses

The Society of Pediatric Nurses (SPN) is the premiere pediatric nursing association advancing the specialty of pediatric nursing through excellence in education, research, and practice. SPN is committed to promoting the care of children and their families through the development of evidence-based standards, visionary leadership, and life-long learning (https://www.pedsnurses.org/).

About the American Pediatric Surgical Nurses Association

The American Pediatric Surgical Nurses Association (APSNA) is the professional association for pediatric surgical nurses. APSNA's mission is that all pediatric surgical patients will receive the highest quality nursing care that is patient and family centered, and its vision is to promote excellence in pediatric surgical nursing practice through educational offerings, nursing research, professional collaboration, and peer support. APSNA has been the leading association for pediatric surgical nursing issues since 1992, providing clinical expertise in this arena both in the outpatient and inpatient setting. Our members include national healthcare experts, authors, researchers, and distinguished faculty and leaders in pediatric surgical care (http://www.apsna.org/).

About the Association of Pediatric Gastroenterology and Nutrition Nurses

The Association of Pediatric Gastroenterology and Nutrition Nurses (APGNN) is a North American organization of nurses and other medical professionals committed to the care of children, and their families, who have gastroenterology/nutrition illnesses. APGNN carries out its mission through the enhancement of professional development and education of patients and caregivers. Since inception in 1989, APGNN has promoted nursing research and education in pediatric gastroenterology and nutrition. APGNN has established standards of pediatric gastroenterology nursing practice while creating a nursing network to enhance professionalism in the discipline. That network continues to support the professional role development of pediatric gastroenterology and nutrition nurses (http://apgnn.org/).

About the Pediatric Endocrinology Nursing Society

The Pediatric Endocrinology Nursing Society (PENS) is committed to the development and advancement of nurses in the art and science of pediatric endocrinology nursing (http://www.pens.org/).

About the Society of Pediatric Cardiovascular Nurses

The Society of Pediatric Cardiovascular Nurses (SPCN) is the only international organization dedicated to expanding nursing knowledge and expertise in the care of children and young adults with heart disease. SPCN members are all involved in the care of children and young adults with congenital heart disease (CHD) and come from almost every state in the United States and eleven countries (http://spcnonline.com).

About the American Nurses Association

The American Nurses Association (ANA) is the only full-service professional organization representing the interests of the nation's 3.4 million registered nurses through its constituent member nurses associations and its organizational affiliates. ANA advances the nursing profession by fostering high standards of nursing practice, promoting the rights of nurses in the workplace, projecting a positive and realistic view of nursing, and by lobbying the Congress and regulatory agencies on healthcare issues affecting nurses and the public.

Preface

In 2008, representatives from the National Association of Pediatric Nurse Practitioners (NAPNAP) and the Society of Pediatric Nurses (SPN) joined with the American Nurses Association (ANA) to produce a unified scope and standards of pediatric nursing practice document for the benefit of children and their families, all the nurses who care for them, and the public at large. Five years later, when the time came to revise the document, NAPNAP and SPN again led the effort, believing it was important, indeed critical, to capture the knowledge and expertise of pediatric specialty organizations. In that effort, they collaborated with the American Pediatric Surgical Nurses Association (APSNA), the Association of Faculties of Pediatric Nurse Practitioners (AFPNP), the Association of Pediatric Gastroenterology and Nutrition Nurses (APGNN), the Pediatric Endocrinology Nursing Society (PENS), and the Society of Pediatric Cardiovascular Nurses (SPCN).

The 2008 publication focused on integrating and updating ground breaking work that was put forth in the original *Scope and Standards of Pediatric Nursing Practice* (ANA & SPN, 2003), *Scope and Standards of Practice: Pediatric Nurse Practitioner (PNP)* (NAPNAP, 2004), as well as *Nursing: Scope and Standards of Practice* (ANA, 2004). By developing a unified document, NAPNAP and SPN sought to reduce confusion and create a new and improved set of standards that addressed all areas of pediatric nursing practice that informed practitioners, the nursing profession, legislators, regulators, accrediting bodies, and the public.

In this 2015 edition, the authors believed that the assumptions specified in the first edition continue to be valid. In the first edition, several assumptions described in the monograph *Changes in Healthcare Professions' Scope of Practice: Legislative Considerations* (NCSBN, 2012) guided the writing. This work, put forth by an interdisciplinary panel of health professional groups, including nursing, social work, medicine, pharmacy, and physical and occupational therapy, suggests the following:

1. Public protection should have top priority in scope of practice decisions.

2. Changes in scope of practice are inherent in the current healthcare system.

3. Collaboration among healthcare providers should be the professional norm.

4. Overlap among professions is necessary.

5. Practice acts should require licensees to demonstrate the training and competence required to provide a service.

No one profession owns a skill or activity in and of itself. Rather, it is the entire scope of activities within a practice that makes a particular profession unique.

Since 2008, the profession of nursing has been called upon to step forward and play a critical role in transforming health care. *The Future of Nursing: Leading Change, Advancing Health* (IOM, 2011) has ignited nursing in ways not seen before; indeed, three of the four key messages in that report underscore the importance of the work that this pediatric nursing scope and standards document represents. Those messages include:

1. Nurses should practice to the full extent of their education and training (p. 29).

2. Nurses should achieve higher levels of education and training through an improved education system that promotes seamless academic progression (p. 30).

3. Nurses should be full partners, with physicians and other health professionals, in redesigning health care in the United States (p. 32).

Pediatric Nursing: Scope and Standards of Practice, Second Edition should be used in conjunction with *Nursing: Scope and Standards of Practice, Second Edition* (ANA, 2010), *Nursing's Social Policy Statement: The Essence of the Profession* (ANA, 2010), *Code of Ethics for Nurses with Interpretive Statements* (ANA, 2015), *Population-Focused Nurse Practitioner Competencies* (NONPF, 2013), and other documents that outline the values, beliefs, and practice of pediatric nurses. *Pediatric Nursing: Scope and Standards of Practice, Second Edition* reflects and guides the practice of pediatric registered nurses and advanced practice registered nurses who provide clinical care to children and their families. It also provides useful information to families and stakeholders such as administrators, educators, policy-makers, and others invested in accessing, delivering, and financing health care. Additionally, the document will provide guidance in evaluating the effectiveness and appropriateness of healthcare delivery in pediatric settings.

Pediatric Nursing: Scope and Standards of Practice, Second Edition describes the scope of activities inherent in pediatric nursing. This one document speaks to the standards of professional performance in all areas of pediatric nursing practice and will serve as a resource not only for nursing faculty and students but also for healthcare providers, researchers, and those involved in funding, legal, policy, and regulatory activities.

Pediatric Nursing: Scope and Standards of Practice, Second Edition will be useful in daily practice and when answering larger questions relating to education, public policy, and advocacy. This resource will reinforce the inclusion of pediatric nursing as an important component in the plans of study for registered nurses. The health of the nation's children is dependent on well-educated, qualified, and competent nurses who have the requisite knowledge and skill to care for the more than 73 million children and adolescents living in the United States today (U.S. Census Bureau, 2010).

This edition introduces or expands upon two areas of importance to nursing: the concept of healthcare transitions and mental health as an area of significance. The population of children with chronic physical, medical, and mental health conditions continues to grow, estimated to be between 10 and 20 million children in the United States (American Academy of Pediatrics, 2013). Both of these topics are now included under *Settings for Pediatric Nursing Practice.*

Finally, the writing committee, after much discussion and feedback from our neonatal nurse practitioner colleagues, removed the neonatal nursing specialty from this edition. This action is entirely appropriate and consistent with the Consensus Model for Advanced Practice Registered Nurse (APRN) Regulation (2008), which specifies the neonatal population as a separate and distinct focus. In 2013, the National Association of Neonatal Nurses, in collaboration with the American Nurses Association, released a second edition of *Neonatal Nursing: Scope and Standards of Practice* that defines the level of nursing practice and professional performance for neonatal nurses at all practice levels and in all settings for the neonatal population.

Creating or revising a document of this nature requires a team of dedicated professionals to move the work forward and produce a scholarly product that will serve the profession, the specialty, and the public. In particular, the chairs would like to acknowledge the members of the writing work group: Cathy Haut, Dolores Jones, and Eileen Arnold of NAPNAP; Lynette Juluke and Mary Lynch of SPN; Jean Ivey of AFPNP; Diane Kocovsky of APGNN; Carmel McComiskey of APSNA; Isabel Couto of PENS; and Mary Rummell of SPCN. This work builds on the distinguished first edition led by Martha K. Swartz (NAPNAP) and Lynn Mohr (SPN). While much of this edition has remained the same, the second edition has added new topics and revised and/ or clarified portions of the scope and standards. A Review Panel Work Group consisting of members of NAPNAP, SPN, AFPNP, APGNN, APSNA, PENS, and SPCN reviewed the draft document. A call for public comment posted on the ANA, NAPNAP, and SPN websites generated review responses. In many ways, the work of writing pediatric nursing's scope and standards of practice is an ongoing process, as the profession and pediatric nursing specialty continue to evolve and the healthcare climate changes. To all who participated in these important steps, thank you!

Patricia Clinton, PhD, RN, CPNP, FAANP, FAAN (Cochair, NAPNAP
Wayne Neal, MAT, BSN, RN-BC (Cochair, SPN)

Introduction

Pediatric nursing focuses on the protection, promotion, and optimization of health and abilities for children from newborn age through young adulthood. Utilizing a patient- and family-centered care approach, pediatric nursing strives for the prevention of illness and injury, the restoration of health, and the maximization of comfort in health conditions and at the end of life, through diagnosis, treatment, and management of the child's condition and advocacy in the care of children and families.

Pediatric nursing has been a specialty since 1855 when the first children's hospital was founded in Philadelphia, Pennsylvania, primarily with a goal of decreasing childhood mortality through research (Taylor, 2006). Over the next 30 years, children's hospitals opened in other major cities, offering opportunities for nurses to care for this specialty population of patients between the ages of birth and 21 years. Managing communicable diseases was one objective of the children's hospital initiative along with offering surgical services, identifying preventative health measures, and providing more sophisticated care. In 1893, a New York City nurse, Lillian Wald, pioneered the new nursing specialty of public health nursing, an important concept of child health (Taylor, 2006).

Pediatric medicine and nursing specialties evolved in response to the presence of children's hospitals and, along with public health goals, the pediatric nursing specialty was established. However, education in pediatric nursing was minimal. The Children's Hospital in Philadelphia opened its own nursing school to provide staff with the necessary knowledge to provide the care, observation, assessment, and education needed by children and their families (Taylor, 2006). Early pediatric nursing focused on improving feeding and preventing illness to decrease mortality rates. This function of pediatric nursing expanded to community programs initiated for the treatment of minor injuries and illnesses and the evolution of social clubs for nurses, leading to schools of nursing in New York in 1902. By 1917, the standard curriculum for schools of nursing included classes on pediatric nursing. The Goldmark Report in 1923 cited nursing education for its failure to provide adequate instruction in public health and pediatric nursing, especially in the prevention of communicable disease, one of the greatest causes of mortality in young children (Taylor, 2006). This strengthened university nursing education programs and directly influenced the move toward advanced degrees and practice.

First-time events in pediatric clinical practice have led to changes in hospital nursing practice. In Boston, the beginnings of modern heart surgery involved children, with the ligation of a patent ductus arteriosus (PDA) in 1938 followed by the creation of an arteriopulmonary shunt (Blalock-Taussig [BT] Shunt) at Johns Hopkins in 1944. Ten years later, more complicated surgical procedures involving bypass circuits required nursing care provided by specialized nurses in specialized units (Noonan, 2004). Responding to the need for community and preventive health services for children, pediatric nurses provided the model for the first nurse practitioner role, developed by Dr. Loretta Ford and Dr. Henry Silver at the University of Colorado in 1964 (Silver, Ford, & Stearly, 1967). Pediatric nurse practitioners (PNPs) now provide care in any settings where children are patients, including acute and critical care.

Pediatric nurses led the movement for family-centered care, currently known as patient- and family-centered care, with research beginning in the 1940s, focusing on the positive effects of involving families in the care of children. Currently, patient- and family-centered care is considered the standard of pediatric health care by many clinical practices, hospitals, and healthcare groups (Kuo et al., 2011). Supported initially by Surgeon General C. Everett Koop's 1987 report, healthcare systems, state and federal governments, and the Institute of Medicine and Healthy People 2020 recognize patient- and family-centered care as integral to patient health, satisfaction, and quality health care. As of 2014, community-based, patient- and family-centered care has expanded to include the care of acute and chronically ill adults as well as children (Kuo et al., 2011).

Today, modern technology has transformed pediatric nursing practice but has required a higher level of knowledge and skill. This challenges the pediatric nurse to develop an ever-evolving technology skill set while continuing to provide cost-effective, efficient care within the philosophy of health promotion, illness and injury prevention, and patient- and family-centered care, regardless of position or setting. To support ongoing learning over the past 30 years, pediatric nurses may choose to acquire certification in general pediatric nursing or a variety of specialties. Pediatric nursing has progressed from a primary hospital base to community and school service settings, with hospitalized children representing the highest level of acuity. These changes have challenged nurse educators and managers to include more in the curriculum and settings with preceptors in order to prepare students for current pediatric nursing. The complexity in technology and skills mandates the need for extensive orientation programs for new nurses regardless of the pediatric practice setting, while at the same time, the high demand for pediatric nurses in the workforce mandates the need for shorter training programs. Modern nurse educators must provide sufficient training to meet the growing needs.

The pediatric population is broadly defined to include all children from birth through 21 years of age and, in specific situations, to individuals older than 21 years until appropriate transition to adult health care is successful (NAPNAP, 2008). Due to improved pediatric care, some populations of young adults now outnumber children with special healthcare needs, chronic conditions, and disabilities such as congenital heart defects. These patients need a plan to transition care from pediatric to adult healthcare settings (Davis, Brown, Taylor, Epstein, & McPheeters, 2014). With an extensive knowledge base regarding developmental issues and concerns of adolescents and young adults, pediatric nurses are qualified to assist youth during the transition phase. Creating an exclusive upper age limit for pediatric patients may unnecessarily create barriers and limit access to health care for this population. In some instances, care continues to be provided in pediatric hospitals, challenging the pediatric nurse to meet the physical and psychosocial needs of adults (Kovacs, 2011; Kim, 2011).

Function of the Scope of Practice Statement

A 1995 Pew Health Professions Commission report (Finocchio et al., 1995, p. ix) defined scope of practice as:

> Definition of the rules, the regulations, and the boundaries within which a fully qualified practitioner with substantial and appropriate training, knowledge, and experience may practice in a field of medicine or surgery, or other specifically defined field. Such practice is also governed by requirements for continuing education and professional accountability.

A nursing scope of practice statement describes the *who, what, where, when, why,* and *how* of nursing practice. Each of these questions must be sufficiently answered to provide a complete picture of the practice, its boundaries, and membership. The depth and breadth in which individual nurses engage in the total scope of nursing practice is dependent upon education, certification, individual states' nursing rules and regulations, experience, organization in which one practices, role, and the population served.

Definition and Function of Standards

Standards are authoritative statements in which the profession, in this case nursing, describes the responsibilities for which its practitioners are accountable. Consequently, standards reflect the values and priorities of the profession.

Standards provide direction for professional nursing education and practice and a framework for evaluation. Written in measurable terms, standards also define the nursing profession's accountability to the public and the practice outcomes for which nurses are responsible.

Development of Standards

Standards of professional nursing practice may pertain to general or specialty practice. Each professional nursing organization has a responsibility to its membership and the public it serves to develop standards of practice. This publication, building upon the standards set forth in the first edition of the *Pediatric Nursing Scope and Standards of Practice*, describes aspects of competent nursing care and professional performance that are measurable, able to be evaluated, and common to nurses engaged in the care of children and their families.

About This Book
Assumptions

Pediatric Nursing: Scope and Standards of Practice, Second Edition focuses primarily on the processes of providing pediatric nursing care at the registered nurse and advanced practice registered nurse levels, and the performance of professional role activities. These standards apply to all nurses involved in the care of children and their families, and they are applicable despite the extensive variability among practice settings. Recognizing the link between the professional work environment and the pediatric nurse's ability to deliver care, employers must provide an environment supportive of nursing practice.

The first major assumption underlying this document is that nursing care is individualized to meet a particular child's or family's unique needs and situation, while focusing on individual, cultural, ethnic, and religious values and beliefs. This includes respect for the goals and preferences of the child and family in developing and implementing a plan of care. Pediatric nurses provide children and their families with individualized information, which empowers them to make informed decisions regarding their health care, including health promotion, prevention of disease, and attainment of a peaceful death.

A second major assumption is that the pediatric nurse establishes a partnership with the child, family, and other healthcare providers. In this partnership, the nurse works collaboratively to coordinate provided care. The degree of participation by the child and family will vary based upon preference, ability, and the child's age, developmental abilities, and cognitive understanding of the care plan.

Organizing Principles

According to *Nursing's Social Policy Statement: The Essence of the Profession* (ANA, 2010), the recipients of nursing care are individuals, groups, families, communities, and populations. *Pediatric Nursing: Scope and Standards of Practice, Second Edition* uses the terms client, patient, child, and family to indicate the person(s) for whom the nurse is providing health care. Care is provided to assist the child or family, sick or well, in performance of those activities contributing to health, recovery, or peaceful death that the child or family would perform unaided if they had the necessary skills, strength, will, or knowledge (Henderson, 1964).

Consideration of the cultural, racial, ethnic, social, economic, and developmental aspects of the child and family is essential to providing nursing services and developing a plan of care. Children's health status must be viewed within the context of their environment and developmental continuum (World Health Organization [WHO] 2007). The International Classification of Functioning, Disability, and Health–Children and Youth Version (ICF–CY) addresses elements of body system and structure functioning, activity limitations, and participation restrictions a child may encounter. Further, environmental factors, specific to the child's immediate surroundings and the more general environment, are also a critical component of the classification scheme (WHO, 2007). Additionally, patients with developmental disabilities are present in all communities and care settings, remaining a vulnerable population. Whatever their age, they and their families need assurance of safe and effective nursing care (Nehring et al., 2004).

Pediatric Nursing: Scope and Standards of Practice, Second Edition addresses the scope of practice for pediatric nursing that applies to all registered nurses (RNs) engaged in the nursing care of children and their families, regardless of clinical specialty, practice setting, or educational preparation. Standards that further define the responsibilities of advanced practice registered nurses (APRNs) working with children and families are also articulated in this document.

Pediatric Nursing Standards

Pediatric Nursing: Scope and Standards of Practice, Second Edition provides 17 Standards that are categorized as 6 Standards of Practice and 11 Standards of Professional Performance.

Standards of Practice

1. Assessment

2. Diagnosis

3. Outcomes Identification

4. Planning

5. Implementation

    5A. Coordination of Care

    5B. Health Teaching and Health Promotion

    5C. Consultation

    5D. Prescriptive Authority and Treatment

6. Evaluation

Standards of Professional Performance

7. Ethics

8. Education

9. Evidence-based Practice and Research

10. Quality of Practice

11. Communication

12. Leadership

13. Collaboration

14. Professional Practice Evaluation

15. Resource Utilization

16. Environmental Health

17. Advocacy

Standards of Practice Further Defined

The six Standards of Practice describe a competent level of nursing care, as demonstrated by the nursing process, including assessment, diagnosis, outcome identification, planning, implementation, and evaluation. The nursing process encompasses all significant actions taken by nurses in providing care to all patients and families, and it forms the foundation for clinical decision-making and the integration of the best research evidence with clinical expertise and patient values (ANA, 2010). Several themes are common to all areas of nursing practice and reflect nursing responsibilities for all children and their families. These themes merit additional attention and include:

- Maintaining a safe environment.
- Providing age-appropriate, culturally and ethnically sensitive care that is patient- and family-centered, efficient, and fiscally responsible.
- Ensuring the implementation of evidence-based clinical findings in the practice setting.
- Ensuring continuity of care.
- Coordinating care across settings and among caregivers.
- Communicating effectively with nurses, other healthcare providers, children, and families.
- Educating children and their families about health practices and treatment modalities.
- Managing and protecting patient health information.

These themes will be reflected in the competencies associated with various standards in this document, although the wording may be different. They are highlighted here because they are fundamental to many of the standards, and because they have emerged as being consistently and significantly influential in nursing practice today.

Standards of Professional Performance Further Defined

The eleven Standards of Professional Performance describe a competent level of behavior in the professional role, including activities related to quality of practice, outcomes measurement, education, communication, ethics, collaboration, research and clinical scholarship, resource utilization, leadership, professional accountability, and advocacy. Advocacy, whether for the individual or the healthcare system, is especially significant because of the unique relationships pediatric nurses develop with children and their families and the responsibilities that pediatric nurses shoulder when caring for them. Pediatric nurses give voice when children and families have no voice; they stand when children and families cannot stand; they act when children and families are most vulnerable. Advocacy extends to the healthcare system in the ways that nurses seek positive changes to improve access to health care, ensure safe practice, and achieve quality outcomes. Within all of the Standards of Professional Performance, the advanced practice registered nurse is accountable for several additional competencies that characterize the advanced practice role. These activities include serving in leadership positions within professional organizations, acting as a role model or mentor to other pediatric nurses, participating in research, and using evidence-based practice processes. All nurses are expected to engage in professional role activities appropriate to their education, position, and practice setting. Ultimately, nurses are accountable to themselves, their patients, and their peers for their professional actions.

Competencies

Pediatric Nursing: Scope and Standards of Practice, Second Edition includes competencies that are key indicators of competent practice for pediatric registered nurses and advanced practice registered nurses. Standards should remain stable over time, as they reflect the philosophical values of the profession. However, competencies may be revised to reflect current nursing practice, education, research, advancements in scientific knowledge and clinical practice, consultations with other healthcare professionals, and individualized family needs.

Throughout this document, terms such as *appropriate, pertinent,* and *realistic* are used. This document cannot account for all possible scenarios that the pediatric nurse might encounter in clinical practice. It is imperative that the pediatric nurse exercise judgment based on education, evidence, and experience in determining what is appropriate, pertinent, or realistic. Further direction may be available from documents such as practice guidelines; agency standards; organization policies, procedures, or protocols; and evidence-based reviews.

Guidelines

Guidelines describe a process of patient-care management that has the potential for improving the quality of clinical decision-making. As systematically developed statements based on available scientific evidence, clinical expertise, and expert opinion, guidelines address the care of specific patient populations or phenomena, whereas standards provide a broad framework for practice. Professional organizations have developed many practice guidelines that are applicable to the pediatric population. Guidelines may be used to provide direction for clinical practice policies, procedures, and protocols.

Summary

Pediatric Nursing: Scope and Standards of Practice, Second Edition delineates the professional responsibilities of registered nurses and advanced practice registered nurses engaged in clinical practice related to children and their families, regardless of setting. *Pediatric Nursing: Scope and Standards of Practice, Second Edition* and other nursing practice guidelines serve as a basis for:

- Quality improvement systems
- Data system development
- Regulatory systems
- Healthcare reimbursement and financing methodologies
- Development and evaluation of nursing service delivery systems and organizational structures
- Certification activities
- Job descriptions and performance appraisals
- Agency policies, procedures, and protocols
- Educational offerings, including basic and advanced nursing programs and continuing education
- Research activities
- Consistency in care
- Professional development
- Global health

In order to serve the public and the nursing profession, pediatric nurses must contribute to the development of standards of practice and evidence-based practice guidelines. Standards and guidelines should be evaluated and revised on an ongoing basis so they can be disseminated and used more effectively to enhance and promote the quality of clinical practice. The dynamic nature of the healthcare environment and the growing body of nursing research provide the impetus and opportunity for nurses to ensure competent clinical practice and promote ongoing professional development that enhances the quality of pediatric nursing care.

Scope of Pediatric Nursing Practice

The scope of practice and roles of the pediatric nurse are diverse and dynamic. The intention of this document is to identify some of the issues and trends that define current roles and to highlight the various roles that have evolved to meet the ever-changing healthcare needs of children and families in diverse settings. The document is not intended to restrict role development, but rather to clarify the scope and foundation of pediatric registered nursing and advanced practice registered nursing and to distinguish between these areas of practice.

Practice Context

There are more than 74 million children and adolescents in the United States, accounting for 24% of the nation's population (U.S. Department of Health and Human Services [U.S. DHHS], 2012). About 90% of these children currently have health insurance. Approximately 20% of children experience special healthcare needs, chronic illnesses, or disabilities. The most prevalent chronic conditions among children are asthma (affecting 9% of children), learning disabilities (affecting 8%), mental and behavioral health problems (6%), and obesity (affecting 18% of children between the ages of 6 and 17 years).

Major threats to all children include accidents, violence, substance abuse, and sexually transmitted infections. Injuries are the leading cause of death among those 1 to 24 years of age, and over 50% of injuries are related to motor vehicle collisions. Ten percent of children between the ages of 0 and 17 are victims of child maltreatment (U.S. DHHS, 2012).

The growing problem of youth violence significantly affects children, families, and communities. In 2011, emergency departments treated more than 700,000 young people aged 10–24 years for nonfatal injuries sustained from assaults (Centers for Disease Control and Prevention [CDC], 2011). The Centers for Disease Control and Prevention's Youth Risk Behavior Survey states that "5.4% of students had carried a weapon (e.g., a gun, knife or club) on school property on at least one day during the 30 days before the survey" (Eaton et al., 2012). Firearms in the home also provide a risk for unintentional injury. Additionally, the threats of terrorism and bioterrorism place further strain on the ability of children and their families to cope with uncertainty.

In the United States, both minorities and the poor experience disparities in access to health care, health-related quality of life, illness, and death. Ten percent of the nation's children are living in poverty (U.S. DHHS, 2012). According to the 2010 U.S. Census, one-third of the population identified themselves as members of racial and ethnic minority groups, which are more likely to be poor. A recent data analysis by the Children's Defense Fund (CDF) from the National Health Interview Survey revealed significant racial and ethnic differences from the effects of healthcare coverage and income on outcomes (CDF, 2010). Among the findings by the CDF are:

- Latino children are almost three times as likely and Black children are almost twice as likely as Caucasian children to be uninsured.

- Among uninsured, Black children are 60% more likely than Caucasian children to have an unmet healthcare need.

- In 2008, 5.6% of Caucasian children, 7.9% of Black children, and 10.2% of Hispanic children had an unmet dental need with twice as many of these children going without a dental encounter in more than two years.

In 2011, the U.S. Department of Health and Human Services indicated that among children, disparities persisted in the rates of infant mortality, asthma, lead poisoning, and obesity. The National Immunization Survey demonstrated that even though immunization rates were at the projected 90% rate or higher among children ages 19–35 months, children below the poverty level still had lower coverage for immunization dosing beyond the first three years of life than children living at or above the poverty level (CDC, 2011a).

Healthcare disparities may affect many aspects of a child's health and development and can have lasting effects throughout adolescence and into adulthood. Because childhood is a time of physical, social, intellectual, and emotional growth, the objectives of pediatric nursing practice must include prevention, early identification, and intervention for health problems that may extend to adulthood. To reduce healthcare disparities, pediatric nurses advocate for and provide quality health care. Additionally, they work with the community and policy-makers to foster awareness of child health inequalities, and they may work with other clinicians and public health officials in coalitions to identify resources and implement and evaluate programs of health care.

Despite access to health insurance, barriers to care and documented unmet needs, such as well child and dental care, still exist. Children represent more than half of all Medicaid recipients. On average, Medicaid covers only about 76% of the cost of care, leading to inadequacies in coverage and profound implications for the future of pediatric health care (Fieldston & Altschuler, 2013). Pediatric nurses are key advocates for families, making policy recommendations and evaluating the effects of healthcare programs through research and education.

Quality and Outcome Guidelines for Nursing of Children and Families

Beginning in 2001, the Expert Panel on Children and Families of the American Academy of Nursing initiated a collaborative process to identify the key standards of excellence in the nursing of children and families (Craft-Rosenberg & Krajicek, 2006). These guidelines were developed by a coalition of pediatric and family nurses representing 12 professional organizations, including SPN and NAPNAP. The 18 guidelines of this "paradigm of excellence" provide a template for clinicians, educators, researchers, and policy-makers to promote, evaluate, and improve the quality of health care provided to children and families (Table 1).

The text *Nursing Excellence for Children and Families* devotes a chapter to each of the guidelines, with each chapter presenting a review and analysis of the evidence pertaining to the guideline as well as implications for practice (Craft-Rosenberg & Krajicek, 2006). Clinicians may apply the guidelines to evaluate and change nursing care in the clinical setting. Educators may use the guidelines for curriculum revision, and researchers may use them as a framework for testing interventions to evaluate effectiveness and outcomes. A consumer version of the guidelines has also been developed so that patients and families may evaluate the quality of care received.

Healthcare Home

The concept *healthcare home* or *medical home* provides a framework to improve access to care and eliminate disparities in medical, mental health, and dental health care for children and families through effective care coordination and case management (Brewer, 2011). This concept advocates for a pediatric healthcare home that is "family-centered, accessible, comprehensive, coordinated, culturally sensitive, compassionate, and focused on the overall well-being of children and families" (NAPNAP, 2009). Healthcare home further asserts that all children should have holistic care where each patient/family has an ongoing relationship with a healthcare professional to ensure optimal health. Qualified healthcare providers (pediatricians, pediatric subspecialists, pediatric nurse practitioners, clinical nurse specialists, and registered nurses) should have a collaborative role in the provision of such care that should be available without barriers to service (NAPNAP, 2009).

TABLE 1. Healthcare Quality and Outcome Guidelines

1. Children and youth have an identified healthcare home.
2. The families of children and youth are partners in decisions, planning, and delivery of care.
3. Family values, beliefs, and preferences are part of care.
4. Family strengths and main concerns are obvious in the care of children and youth.
5. Children, youth, and families will have accessible health care.
6. Pregnant women will have accessible health care.
7. Family needs are identified and services offered.
8. Children, youth, and families are directed to community services when needed.
9. Children, youth, and families receive care that promotes and maintains health and prevents disease.
10. Pregnant women, children, youth, and families have access to genetic testing and advice.
11. Children and youth receive care that is physically and emotionally safe.
12. Children's, youth's, and families' privacy and rights are protected.
13. Children and youth who are very ill receive the full range of needed services.
14. Children and youth with disabilities and/or special healthcare needs receive the full range of services.
15. Children, youth, and families receive comfort care.
16. Children's, youths', and families' health and risky behaviors and problems are identified and addressed.
17. Children, youth, and families receive care that supports development.
18. Children, youth, and families are fully informed of the outcomes of care.

Craft-Rosenberg, M., & Krajicek, M. (2006). *Nursing excellence for children and families.* New York, NY: Springer Publishing Co.

The elements of the healthcare or medical home can historically be traced back to public health nursing and the community mental health movement that offered guidelines for providing care to the underserved (American Public Health Association, 1955; Caplan, 1961; Pridham, 1993). Nursing has continued to be a driving force in the development of innovative models for providing high-quality health care, including school-based health centers (SBHCs) and community health centers. Because nurses interact with children and families at multiple entry points in the healthcare system, they play a key role in implementing the healthcare home concept and assuring that care is accessible, comprehensive, continuous, and culturally competent. According to Cowell and Swartwout (2006), nursing care excellence in implementing the healthcare home concept is achieved by:

- Supporting the delivery of care via interdisciplinary teams.
- Creating effective communication and partnerships with each family.
- Enabling global access by providers to healthcare records.
- Involving family members and individualizing care.
- Being an expert at knowing community resources.
- Being an expert on state and federal policies, regulations, and programs.
- Implementing a quality monitoring system.
- Promoting and monitoring preventive care.
- Providing comprehensive primary care.
- Providing creative solutions for those who are uninsured.
- Providing support during periods of transition.
- Working with families with special needs.
- Assisting families in becoming independent, informed consumers of health care.
- Generating nursing research related to the healthcare home concept.

Patient- and Family-centered Care

Patient- and family-centered care is an approach to the planning, delivery, and evaluation of health care that is grounded in mutually beneficial partnerships among healthcare providers, patients, and families. It redefines the relationships in health care. The original definition of patient-centered care, as discussed in the literature in the late 1980s and early 1990s, did not include the concept of patients and families as advisors and essential partners in improving care practices and systems of care. Patients and families influence, change, and move the direction of healthcare systems to improve and enhance the safety and quality of healthcare outcomes across the continuum (Institute for Patient- and Family-Centered Care, 2010).

The majority of patients have some connection to family or support networks and it is important for the health system to encourage the continuing link to these natural supports. The word "family" refers to two or more persons who are related in any way—biologically, legally, or emotionally. The term *family-centered* is not intended to remove control from patients who are competent to make decisions concerning their own health care. In pediatrics, particularly with infants and young children, the patient's parents or guardians define family members. Table 2 outlines the key elements.

Hospitals, clinics, and other healthcare agencies that make an explicit commitment to patient- and family-centered care develop policies, programs, and practices collaboratively with patients and families that support and encourage family presence and participation (Institute for Patient- and Family-Centered Care, 2010). Pediatric nurses embrace and employ the core concepts of patient- and family-centered care. These concepts (Institute for Patient- and Family-Centered Care, 2010) include:

- **Respect and dignity.** Healthcare practitioners listen to and honor patient and family perspectives and choices. Patient and family knowledge, values, beliefs, and cultural backgrounds are incorporated into the planning and delivery of care.

- **Information Sharing.** Healthcare practitioners communicate and share complete and unbiased information with patients and families in ways that are affirming and useful. Patients and families receive timely, complete, and accurate information in order to effectively participate in care and decision-making.

- **Participation.** Patients and families are encouraged and supported in participating in care and decision-making at the level they choose.

- **Collaboration.** Patients and families are also included on an institution-wide basis. Healthcare leaders collaborate with patients and families in policy and program development, implementation, and evaluation; in healthcare facility design; and in professional education, as well as in the delivery of care.

To date, nursing organizations have collaborated with healthcare stakeholders to develop standards and position statements that include the overall importance of the patient experience and patient- and family-centered care concepts. Professional nurses play a vital role in empowering patients and families and have engaged patients and families in their own care for many years.

Evidence-based Practice

Findings reported by the Institute of Medicine (2001) in *Crossing the Quality Chasm: A New Health System for the 21st Century* have challenged all healthcare professionals to deliver care that is based upon the best scientific evidence available, but the gap between publication of research findings and translation of these findings remains a concern. Evidence-based practice (EBP) has been

TABLE 2. Key Elements of Family-centered Care

Key components of family-centered practice include:

- Working with the family unit to ensure the safety and well-being of all family members.

- Strengthening the capacity of families to function effectively by focusing on solutions.

- Engaging, empowering, and partnering with families throughout the decision- and goal-making processes.

- Developing a relationship between parents and service providers characterized by mutual trust, respect, honesty, and open communication.

- Providing individualized, culturally responsive, flexible, and relevant services for each family.

- Linking families with collaborative, comprehensive, culturally relevant, community-based networks of supports and services.

From U.S. DHHS, Child Welfare Information Gateway. (n.d.). "Philosophy and Key Elements of Family-Centered Practice." Retrieved from www.childwelfare.gov/famcentered/philosophy.cfm.

defined as "the integration of best research evidence with clinical expertise and patient values" (Sackett, Straus, Richardson, Rosenberg, & Haynes, 2000). Currently, EBP nursing centers have been developed within universities as well as hospital settings. Moreover, with the advent of the Doctor of Nursing Practice (DNP) degree, evidence-based practice is a key concept in curricula and is identified as one of the eight essentials of DNP education (American Association of Colleges of Nursing, 2006).

Increasingly, clinical practice guidelines developed by professional organizations or expert panels promote the translation of evidence-based findings into nursing care (Melnyk & Fineout-Overholt, 2010). Pediatric nurses acknowledge the need for evidence-based practice in the clinical setting and recognize that continuing research, including research involving children, will be required to gather that evidence. Pediatric nurses advocate for research that involves minimal threat to the child and where potential benefits outweigh risks. Pediatric nurses promote research conducted in a respectful, ethical manner in the hope that findings will benefit the children involved in the studies and the future care of children (SPN, 2004). NAPNAP's outlined research agenda focuses on areas of child concern such as obesity, safety, self-management of illness, mental health, and health promotion (NAPNAP, 2008).

Differentiated Areas of Pediatric Nursing Practice

Pediatric registered nurses and advanced practice registered nurses are licensed nurses who provide health care to children. Specific areas of practice within pediatric nursing are described below.

Pediatric Registered Nurse

The pediatric registered nurse is a licensed nurse who has demonstrated clinical skills and knowledge within pediatrics. The Pediatric Nursing Certification Board (PNCB) and the American Nurses Credentialing Center (ANCC) offer pediatric nursing certification. Many nurses who contribute to the care of children and their families are also responsible for adhering to practice standards as designated by their chosen specialty. Certifications in specialty pediatric areas are available to these nurses.

In 1998, SPN first identified standards for pediatric professional nursing development (Woodring & Pridham, 1998). The competencies focus on the education of the novice nurse and include:

- The unique anatomical, physiological, and developmental differences among neonates, infants, children, adolescents, and young adults in transition.

- Care of children in the context of their families.

- Sensitivity to cultural issues, especially those related to how the family and healthcare providers tend to children's healthcare needs.

- Effective communication with children, families, other healthcare providers, and appropriate educational agency staff.

- Safety assurance and injury prevention for children and their families.

- Promotion of children's health in the context of their families.

- Assessment of the unique growth and development needs of children who have chronic conditions, and of their families.

- Exceptional needs of children with episodic injuries or illnesses.

- Economic, social, and political influences outside the family that have an impact on children's health and development and family functioning.

- Ethical, moral, and legal dilemmas involving children, families, and healthcare professionals.

Pediatric Advanced Practice Registered Nurse

Advanced practice registered nurses are registered nurses who have completed an accredited graduate-level education program, acquired advanced clinical knowledge and skills to provide direct care to patients, and, if required by their state practice act, passed a national certification exam. They build upon the competencies of RNs by demonstrating a greater depth and breadth of knowledge, a strong ability to synthesize data and employ critical thinking, increased complexity of skills and interventions, and significant role autonomy (APRN, 2008). The APRN role combines both specialization and expansion through in-depth study of the research-based, theoretical, and clinical practice issues unique to the specialty population.

In pediatric nursing, the predominant advanced practice roles are the pediatric clinical nurse specialist, the primary care pediatric nurse practitioner, and the acute care pediatric nurse practitioner. These advanced practice registered nurses hold a minimum of a master's degree in pediatric nursing, have attained certification in the advanced practice role, and hold the appropriate credentials as determined by state boards of nursing. The pediatric APRN provides care in an expanded role that incorporates comprehensive assessment skills, diagnostic ability, critical thinking, independent decision-making, collaborative management of health and illness problems, leadership within complex systems, and the ability to critically analyze and translate research findings into practice. APRNs in other clinical settings, such as family practice, nurse midwifery, and nurse anesthesia, are also expected to incorporate advanced knowledge of pediatric concepts into their clinical practice since their client populations may include pediatric patients and their families.

The advanced practice pediatric nursing roles are differentiated from one another by virtue of their unique blend of nursing knowledge, science, and patient population. The following descriptions further illustrate the advanced practice roles that require knowledge specialization and clinical expertise in the care of children and their families.

Pediatric Clinical Nurse Specialist (PCNS)

The PCNS is an APRN prepared as a clinical expert in the specialty of pediatric nursing who, in addition to providing direct patient care, serves as a leader in education, research, quality improvement, outcome monitoring, and consultation with other nurses, health team members, and the community. Clinical nurse specialists are prepared at the master's or doctoral level. CNSs traditionally work for healthcare institutions, but they may also work independently in private or collaborative practice. The National Association of Clinical Nurse Specialists (NACNS) has published a position statement on CNS education and practice in which they identify core CNS competencies and the corresponding core areas of knowledge that should be included in CNS graduate programs (NACNS, 2010). These principal knowledge areas are expanded from the core areas identified in the American Association of Colleges of Nursing's *Essentials of Master's Education for Advanced Practice Nursing* (2011), which documents and includes theoretical foundations, inquiry skills, and empirical and practical knowledge that focus on phenomena of concern, nursing therapeutics, evaluation methodologies, and systems thinking.

Pediatric Nurse Practitioner (PNP)

The PNP provides comprehensive health care to children from birth through young adulthood by assessment, diagnosis, management, and evaluation of care. In accordance with state licensure and regulatory mechanisms, PNPs provide a wide range of pediatric healthcare services in a variety of primary and specialty healthcare settings emphasizing health promotion, injury and disease prevention, and chronic illness management. The PNP may consult with other members of the healthcare team, coordinate care, and make referrals to other healthcare providers. Additionally, the PNP may function as a resource in areas of expertise to colleagues in health professions and other disciplines.

The PNP assumes accountability for professional actions and incorporates risk management strategies into clinical practice. Historically, PNPs have practiced predominantly in primary care settings in which the emphasis is on providing health care that is accessible, comprehensive in scope, and coordinated with specialty practices and community resources in order to maximize continuity. Certification as a PNP, with an emphasis on primary care, is offered by both the Pediatric Nursing Certification Board (PNCB) and the American Nurses Credentialing Center (ANCC) and is required for recognition in most states. The APRN Consensus Model (2008) reflects aspects of the primary and acute care PNP roles related to the population focus. The majority of states support the consensus model and require that PNPs take a pediatric certification examination based on educational preparation in order to be fully licensed by the state (Hartigan, 2011).

The acute care PNP provides cost-effective, quality care for acutely, critically, and chronically ill children who may be experiencing life-threatening illnesses and organ dysfunction or failure. Similar to the primary care PNP, the acute care PNP manages direct patient care within a collaborative practice model, including performing in-depth physical assessments, ordering and interpreting results of laboratory and diagnostic tests, ordering medications, and performing therapeutic procedures in a variety of contexts such as inpatient and outpatient hospital units, emergency departments, and home care settings. The foundation of advanced practice nursing also provides general role expectations for the acute care PNP, which include expertise in patient care that is based on clinical evidence and theory, progressive leadership, and involvement in education and research.

The role of the acute care PNP began to evolve in the late 1990s, as nurse practitioner practice expanded into critical care units, specialty practice sites, and emergency departments. The expansion of the role was also in keeping with recommendations of the Institute of Medicine, which called for a greater commitment to interdisciplinary care (2001). The increased demand for PNPs with the knowledge and skills necessary for acute care practice led to progressive changes in the education of PNPs for this role. NAPNAP developed a position statement for the acute care PNP (NAPNAP, 2010). Similarly, the National Panel for Acute Care Nurse Practitioner Competencies, in collaboration with the Association of Faculties of Pediatric Nurse Practitioners (AFPNP), developed a set of core competencies for PNPs in acute care (2004), which was replaced by NP competencies specific to the population focus in 2013 (National Organization of Nurse Practitioner Faculties, 2013). These competencies provide the basis for curriculum development, evaluation, and certification. The Pediatric Nursing Certification Board (PNCB) offers certification for the acute care PNP requiring graduation from an accredited acute care PNP program.

Regulatory Challenges for Advanced Practice Registered Nurses

All nurse practitioners and clinical nurse specialists function according to their state Nurse Practice Act and in accordance with individual state laws and regulations. States vary in their regulations, including the granting of prescriptive privileges, and specific state requirements must be recognized and met. Twenty-one states and the District of Columbia have granted advanced practice nurses full practice authority (AANP, May 2015). In some states, however, impediments to the full use of advanced practice registered nurses include:

- Legal barriers such as laws that require physician supervision or limit an advanced practice registered nurse's prescriptive authority.

- Financial barriers that prevent public and private payers from reimbursing advanced practice registered nurses.

- Professional barriers.

Advanced practice registered nurses practice across all settings and patient populations and provide coordinated and cost-effective care but there remain significant "regulatory obstacles and restrictions that currently impede the full realization of their potential" (Institute Of Medicine, 2011, p. 444). The IOM report recommends that nurses function to the fullest extent of their education and training and be full partners with physicians and other healthcare professionals in redesigning health care. Healthcare regulatory organizations have acknowledged that it is not reasonable to expect each health profession to have a unique scope of practice, and that there is considerable overlap among the abilities and skill sets of each discipline (National Council of State Boards of Nursing, 2009). Scope of practice changes should reflect the evolution of the abilities of practitioners within a healthcare discipline to provide care in a safe and effective manner in order to better protect the public and enhance consumer access to quality health care.

The increased focus on interprofessional practice to deliver health care, supported by the 2011 Institute of Medicine report *The Future of Nursing* and the 2010 Patient Protection and Affordable Care Act (U.S. DHHS, 2013) emphasizing primary care and health insurance for the uninsured, is important to the nursing profession and the pediatric specialty. These two references call for more nurses and APRNs to function with greater autonomy and be recognized for their contributions to health care.

Caring for a Diverse Population

It is fundamental that nursing practice provides culturally sensitive and competent care that values diversity, is based on self-assessment, and effectively manages the dynamic differences between individuals and groups. Due to the expanding cultural diversity of the American population, pediatric nurses must have working knowledge of the cultural characteristics and practices of the most-served population in their clinical areas, while remaining aware of their own personal values and beliefs. Understanding cultural views can help the pediatric nurse anticipate and understand why and how families make certain decisions regarding their child's health. Cultural and religious beliefs and practices can affect the management of the ill child, so pediatric nurses must incorporate them into the child and family care plan. It is imperative for pediatric nurses to apply knowledge of and demonstrate respect for culture and religion as a framework in the provision of care. When necessary, however, they should seek additional resources and make adjustments when beliefs and practices are unsafe for the child.

An appreciation of diversity and the promotion of inclusivity are also important when providing care to youth who are gay, lesbian, bisexual, transgender, or questioning their sexual orientation/gender identity (GLBTQ). Many GLBTQ youth encounter prejudice, stigma, hostility, or hatred that may hinder their ability to achieve developmental tasks. These children tend to experience higher levels of isolation, runaway behavior, homelessness, domestic violence, depression, anxiety, suicide, violent victimization, substance abuse, and school or job failure than heterosexual or gender-conforming youth (Chaplic & Allen, 2013). Pediatric nurses should individualize interventions relating to health promotion and risk reduction for youth who identify or are struggling with identifying themselves as GLBTQ (NAPNAP, 2011).

Healthcare Transitions

The concept of healthcare transition was originally described as the "purposeful, planned movement of adolescents and young adults with chronic physical and medical conditions from child-centered to adult-oriented healthcare systems with the optimal goal of providing health care that is uninterrupted, coordinated, developmentally appropriate, psychologically sound and comprehensive" (Blum et al., 1993, p. 570–76). Transitional care is an organized effort to provide pediatric patients with the tools and resources they need to assume personal responsibility for their medical care while facilitating their transfer from a pediatric care provider to an adult practitioner (Philpott, 2011). Healthcare transition is an increasingly recognized area of importance (Crowley, Wolfe, Lock, & McKee, 2011).

Advances in medical treatments and technologies have led to improved long-term outcomes for adolescents and young adults with special healthcare needs, chronic conditions, and disabilities (Fernandes et al., 2014). Transitioning the growing population of adolescents with chronic medical illnesses to adult healthcare providers is an important yet challenging element of medical care, currently recognized as a model of care requiring a transition plan (AAP, 2011). Disciplines with larger proportions of pediatric patients with chronic diseases, including cystic fibrosis, hematological disease, diabetes mellitus, organ transplant, and congenital heart disease, have conducted significant amounts of research regarding transitional care (Philpott, 2011).

Two national surveys of children with special healthcare needs indicate limited achievement of national health policy goals for transition, which were determined in 2002 (U.S. DHHS, 2004, 2008). The U.S. Department of Health and Human Services Maternal and Child Health Bureau has outlined a six-step procedure for successful transition to adult care. These six steps include initiating a transition policy, maintaining a patient registry of those who will soon be ready for adult providers, assessing readiness, planning the actual transition, and creating a transition completeness plan in which pediatric providers will continue communication with adult healthcare providers for a period of three months following the transition (Center for Healthcare Transition Improvement, 2012). Pediatric nurses are in a unique position to play an active role in the process of transition. APRNs have traditionally focused on wellness and management of acute common childhood illnesses in the primary care setting. APRNs and pediatric nurses require the skills needed to develop interventions focusing on the improvement of health and safety of children with special healthcare needs as they transition to adult care (Looman, O'Connor-Von, & Lindeke, 2008).

The passage from adolescence to adulthood is a time of internal turmoil and rapid change (Lemly, Weitzman, & O'Hare, 2013). For chronically ill adolescents, the transition to adulthood is especially stressful for the child, family, and the healthcare providers involved in the transfer to adult care (AAP, American Academy of Family Physicians, & American College of Physicians, 2011). Pediatric nurses and APRNs are responsible for planning the transfer, accommodating for the adolescent's long-term needs. The pediatric nurse must possess a clear understanding of the transition process and actively help to develop strategies needed to support patients and families through this process. An awareness of some of the relevant issues pertaining to adolescent transitions, especially those related to health care, is essential. The pediatric nurse needs to develop processes for collaborating with their adolescent patients, families, and other professionals to facilitate successful transitions to healthier, productive, and satisfying adulthoods (Fernandes et al., 2014).

A well-planned transition from child to adult health care requires individual planning and coordination of patient, family, and provider responsibilities (AAP, 2011). As they become adults, adolescents evolve from being dependent on their family to becoming independently responsible for their own medical care (Leung, Heyman, & Mahadevan, 2011). The pediatric nurse should provide educational resources to help chronically ill adolescents develop the necessary skills to manage their care as independent adults, introducing the concept of transfer to adult care in advance and developing communication routes to facilitate the transfer from pediatric to adult care providers (Philpott, 2011). Adolescents transitioning to an adult healthcare system require skills in communication, decision-making, personal care, assertiveness, self-determination, and advocacy (Hait & Fishman, 2006). A successful transition from a pediatric to an adult provider will allow the patient to acquire these skills and ensure continuity of age-appropriate health care between different providers.

Settings for Pediatric Nursing Practice: Pediatric Registered Nurse and Advanced Practice Registered Nurse

Practice settings for pediatric nurses and advanced practice registered nurses are multiple and varied. Setting locations include hospitals, homes, community organizations, clinics, schools, and camps. A pediatric registered nurse or advanced practice registered nurse may direct care that is acute, chronic, or palliative/hospice.

Children's hospitals are not isolated units or buildings, but provide services to all children in their communities through urgent and emergency care, primary care, wellness promotion, injury prevention, child abuse prevention, and community/school health services. In the United States, there are 50–55 freestanding/independent children's hospitals, 110–125 children's hospitals as part of a larger hospital medical system, including academic medical centers and community hospitals, and 90–100 specialized children's hospitals, including burns, orthopedic, rehabilitation, and psychiatry. In 2011, freestanding/independent children's hospitals saw approximately 2.4 million emergency patients and 12 million outpatients. These children's hospitals provide 99% of all pediatric organ transplants, 92% of all pediatric cardiac surgical care, and 89% of all pediatric cancer care. In the United States, there are only four Shriner's Hospitals that provide 72% of all burn beds and services, and 10 specialty hospitals that provide 52% of all pediatric rehabilitation beds and services (Children's Hospital Association, 2013). These hospitals provide the training for the nation's pediatric specialists and provide the setting in which to conduct research on the cures for diseases that affect children.

Many children's hospitals have set up networks to market their expertise to community facilities locally and by tele-medicine, improving access to specialized health care. This allows children with low-acuity care requirements to remain in facilities closer to home and allows freestanding/independent children's hospitals or facilities within academic medical centers to treat children who require higher-acuity, specialized care.

Inpatient and Acute Care Settings
The biomedical advances that are available to adult patients with acute and chronic conditions are also available to pediatric patients. New technologies, including monitoring equipment, specialized assessment tools, and complex intervention modalities, are available for neonates and children as well as adults. Pediatric nurses are proficient in the use of resuscitation equipment, home and multimode ventilators, artificial airways including tracheostomies, dialysis (both hemo and peritoneal), ventricular assist devices, hyper/hypothermia management, intravenous therapy, venous/arterial/intracranial pressure monitoring, feeding pumps, diabetic management tools, acute and chronic pain management, and other specialized technologies. The pediatric nurse must maintain a safe patient environment while using the complex technology.

Pediatric Home Healthcare Settings
Technological advances have made the home care of children with complex, chronic diseases and congenital conditions possible. Many home healthcare agencies employ skilled pediatric nurses to care for medically fragile children with multiple technological and nursing care needs. These children may have tracheostomies, require home ventilators or respiratory assist devices, need

continuous parenteral or gastric feedings, rely on peritoneal dialysis, receive multiple intravenous medications, have frequent and complex dressing changes, or may even have a ventricular assist device for cardiac output.

Pediatric nurses practicing in home health care address the environmental, social, and personal factors affecting health and may provide care that family or friends cannot offer on a consistent basis. Medication management, fall prevention, infection prevention, and safe patient hand-offs are critically important for the pediatric patient. The role of the pediatric nurse in transitioning these inpatients to home is complex and the key to successful home management. The nurse must have educator skills to teach the family/caregiver and evaluate their comprehension and the quality of care provided. The focus of home health care is on preventing admission to an acute care setting, offering assistance to families, and providing direct treatment in the home. This specialized care requires a pediatric nurse who provides developmentally appropriate, patient- and family-centered, atraumatic care with advanced knowledge of the technology needed by this unique population.

Perioperative and Surgical Settings

Pediatric surgical nursing involves care for children throughout the surgical experience, including: preoperative preparation and teaching, inpatient and outpatient intraoperative care, and postoperative care for procedures such as major or minimally invasive surgery, innovative therapies, fetal surgery, and pediatric solid organ transplantation. Perioperative nurses provide direct patient care, coordinate the multidisciplinary surgical care team, and provide emotional and psychosocial support to the family and child. The American Pediatric Surgical Nurses Association (APSNA) is the specialty organization for those pediatric nurses involved in perioperative nursing.

Hospice and Palliative Care Settings

The statistics regarding pediatric chronic illness and mortality are staggering. According to the National Center for Health Statistics, over 53,000 children in the United States die each year and over 2 million children live with a chronic illness (CDC, 2011b). The number of pediatric deaths is small compared to the 2.5 million adult deaths each year, so the emphasis of care from both financial and educational objectives has been focused on the adult population. Because of advances in medicine, over 400,000 children now live with chronic disabling conditions and could benefit from palliative care (National Hospice and Palliative Care Organization, 2012). Despite an increased awareness of the need for palliative care services for children, the majority of children who die have not had the benefit of these services (AAP, 2012). Pediatric palliative and/or hospice care (PP/HC) is both a philosophy and an organized method for delivering competent, compassionate, and consistent care to children with chronic, complex, and/or life-threatening conditions and their families. This care focuses on enhancing quality of life, minimizing suffering, optimizing function, and providing opportunities for personal and spiritual growth (National Hospice and Palliative Care Organization, 2012).

Planned and delivered through the collaborative efforts of an interdisciplinary team with the child, family, and caregivers at its center, PP/HC can and should be provided along with concurrent disease-modifying therapy or as the focus of care. PP/HC is achieved through a combination of active and compassionate therapies intended to comfort and support the child, his or her family members, and other significant people in the child's life. Effective management of pain and other distressing symptoms, together with psychosocial and spiritual care, are of critical importance from diagnosis through the entire course of a child's life. Therapies take a holistic approach, assisting children and families in fulfilling their physical, psychological, educational, social, and spiritual goals while remaining sensitive to developmental, personal, cultural, and religious values, beliefs, and practices.

PP/HC differs from palliative and/or hospice care delivered to adults in several important ways. People with palliative care needs range in age from prenatal babies to adults with conditions, followed by pediatric subspecialists, or those whose developmental and/or physical challenges are better served by pediatric care providers. PP/HC teams must thus be able to care for a wide range of patients whose understanding of illness and decision-making changes significantly throughout the developmental spectrum. Pediatric trajectories of illness, clinical models of care delivery, funding mechanisms, research paradigms, educational initiatives, communication strategies, ethical concerns, staffing ratios, and effective pain and symptom management interventions are all significantly different from those effective for adult patients (AAP, 2012; National Hospice and Palliative Care Organization, 2012).

Ambulatory Care Settings

Ambulatory care settings offer children and their families, especially those with chronic conditions, the opportunity to develop ongoing relationships with healthcare professionals. As a result, the pediatric nurse in this setting can develop a mutually gratifying, therapeutic relationship with the child and family. This long-term relationship can provide a more complete picture of the child's general well-being and ability to achieve developmental milestones. Illness prevention and health promotion activities are the core interventions of the nurse and the healthcare team. For children coping with a chronic condition, the healthcare team also focuses on maintaining optimum levels of health for the child.

The nurse practicing in a specialty pediatric clinic collaborates with an inter-professional team to meet the challenges of patients with chronic or terminal illnesses. Quality health care for these children often requires significant case coordination so that the care provided is accessible, comprehensive, continuous, and efficient. Throughout the care process, the nurse serves as a vital link in the communication between health team members and the family.

Community Health and School Settings

Community health settings provide the pediatric nurse an opportunity to affect large populations of children and families positively through community health organizations, schools, and city and state departments of health. Many community health programs are aimed at prevention, education, and provision of programs, such as immunizations and screening.

Pediatric school nurses work in public or private school systems, or in county, city, or state governmental agencies. The National Association of School Nurses (NASN) promotes the need for access to school nurses and has a position statement outlining the need for school nurses in caring for chronically ill children (NASN, 2012). The school nurse is often responsible for meeting the needs of children in more than one school and ideally works with aides, health associates, and/or other unlicensed assistive personnel who are responsible for monitoring day-to-day school health problems. The school nurse is responsible for overall management and delegation of activities to the aides and for evaluating the appropriateness of interventions provided to ailing children.

School nursing is a specialized practice of professional nursing that advances the well-being, academic success, and lifelong achievement of students. The educational requirements for school nurses vary from state to state; however, the NASN recommends a baccalaureate degree in nursing from an accredited college or university and licensure as a registered nurse as the minimal preparation necessary to enter school nursing practice (NASN, 2012). School nurses work with the students, parents or guardians, healthcare practitioners, teachers, school administrators, and other professionals in the school setting and the community to provide or secure health services for children.

School nurses need to have expertise in clinical nursing, communication, surveillance, education, advocacy, and leadership in order to ensure that all students' health needs are addressed. The school nurse's role includes assessing the health status of students, identifying problems that have an impact on health and learning, delivering emergency care, administering medications, performing healthcare procedures, providing wellness programs, advocating for children and families, and providing health counseling and education. School nurses may be first responders for infectious disease outbreaks and episodes of violence or bioterrorism within and around the school. Overall, school nursing involves planning, developing, managing, and evaluating healthcare services to children in an educational setting, and encompasses working with the families of the students and the community in which the student resides (Guilday, 2000; NASN & ANA, 2011). School nurses also have their own scope and standards of practice published by ANA and NASN (2011).

Rosenblum and Sprague-McRae (2013) discuss the importance of extending initiatives to increase quality and safety in school nurse continuing education offerings. State funding for school nursing has diminished because of declining state revenues and an increase in alternative private or voucher payment plans leading to decreased public school enrollment.

School-based health centers (SBHCs) provide comprehensive physical and mental health services to children and adolescents, with legal guardianship involvement, at locations accessible to them. SBHCs are not designed to replace an ongoing relationship a child may have with a primary provider, nor to replace the services of a school nurse. Rather, the SBHCs are designed to overcome existing social and economic barriers that prevent access to quality health care. Ideally, students receive comprehensive primary care, including social services, mental health, and health education focused on wellness. Care is delivered in the context of family and community, so that the students may derive maximum benefit from their education (NAPNAP, 2012). SBHCs should meet standards of care similar to those of community health centers, including certification and credentialing processes and a systematic evaluation of service outcomes. In 2012, approximately 790,000 children were served by SBHCs (U.S. DHHS/HRSA, 2013).

A pediatric nurse practitioner and a clinic assistant or receptionist usually staff SBHCs, with access to a team of health educators, physicians, nutritionists, nurses, and social workers. The staff members are prepared to deal with the unique growth, social, developmental, and emotional needs of the school-age population they serve. Activities of the school nurse or clinic may also include sponsoring health fairs and immunization programs, ongoing participation in crisis intervention teams, class health education, parent education, teacher training, sports medicine clinics, student health clubs, question-and-answer columns in student newspapers, involvement in dropout prevention initiatives, and assessing health risk behaviors of the student population.

Pediatric nurses also provide health consultation to early care and education (ECE) programs (Hanna et al., 2012). The role of the childcare health consultant (CCHC) is to minimize health risks and promote healthy behaviors in out-of-home care programs, and to link families with community-based health and developmental services (AAP & APHA, 2011). Specifically, CCHCs promote health practices in ECE programs that may focus on nutrition, safe food handling, infection control, infant sleep position, monitoring of immunizations, and safe and active play. Evidence is emerging that the role of the CCHC can improve overall childcare quality and school readiness among children (AAP & APHA, 2011).

Camp Settings

Camp nursing affords the pediatric nurse the opportunity to provide all aspects of health care in an outdoor setting to either the general pediatric population or a specialty population, such as children with cancer, cystic fibrosis, asthma, diabetes, or developmental disabilities. The primary goal of specialty camps is to allow children, who may have extensive medical treatments or unpleasant life experiences, to enjoy real camping while also learning about their illness or disability. Experienced pediatric nurses with current basic life support and first aid training may choose to practice in camp settings. The Association of Camp Nurses has published *Standards and Scope of Camp Nursing Practice, Second Edition* (ACN, 2005).

Transport Settings

Neonates, children, and adolescents with increased acute care needs and technological support requirements may need air or surface transport from a trauma site, community hospital, or birth hospital to a facility with tertiary intensive capabilities including neonatal and/or pediatric intensive care or other subspecialty units. Pediatric specialty teams are typically composed of two RNs, an RN and APRN, an RN and a physician, or an RN with a physician and a respiratory therapist. The Air and Surface Transport Nurses Association (ASTNA) is a professional association for nurses working in transport settings.

Specialty Settings for Pediatric Advanced Practice Registered Nurses

With continued blending of inpatient and outpatient services, the advanced practice registered nurse provides care in many specific, specialty areas including, but not limited to: cardiology, cardiac surgery, endocrinology, nephrology, neurology/neurosurgery, pediatric surgery and urology, pain/sedation, and palliative/end-of-life care. The APRN provides direct patient care, such as diagnosis treatment planning, consultation, admission privileges, and discharge responsibilities, depending on their individual state licensure. He or she may develop and manage specific programs of care involving growth and developmental assessment, post-op surgical follow-up, management of chronic illnesses, and high-risk clinics for frequent, ongoing assessment, management, and referral. Education programs to support the specialty APRN vary in the scope and breadth of didactic coursework and clinical experiences. Some programs award a master's or doctoral degree with an area of specialization. Others offer a fellowship or post-master's certificate in a specific specialty.

Trends and Issues in Pediatric Nursing
Global Perspectives of Pediatric Nursing

With the increasing ease at which people can travel worldwide, many opportunities exist for pediatric nurses globally. Many nurses travel to underdeveloped countries as part of their undergraduate and graduate educational preparation. Working in clinics, providing education and care to children and families, or serving as medical personnel for missionary teams are just some of the opportunities available to the pediatric registered nurse and advanced practice registered nurse. Through the International Council of Nursing (ICN), pediatric nurses can engage in or support larger global issues, such as quality nursing care for all, sound global health policies, the advancement of nursing knowledge, and the presence worldwide of a respected nursing profession and a competent and satisfied nursing workforce. While advances have been made in recent years in the fulfillment of children's rights to survival, health, and education, these gains are in danger of reversal in some parts of the world. On a global level, the predominant current risks to children are those stemming from poverty, environmental hazards, armed conflict, infectious diseases, and gender inequality (Oberg, 2012).

Complementary Therapies

Increasingly, Americans are turning toward the use of complementary and alternative medicine (CAM) for themselves and their children. CAM is defined as a group of diverse medical and healthcare systems, practices, and products that are not presently considered part of conventional medicine (National Center for Complementary and Alternative Medicine [NCCAM], 2013). This integrative approach combines conventional treatments with those for which there is high-quality evidence of safety and effectiveness. Examples of complementary and alternative therapies include: mind–body techniques (meditation, prayer, creative expression through art, music, or dance), acupuncture, dietary supplements, herbal products, and manipulative or body-based practices such as massage, therapeutic touch, healing touch, Reiki, and magnetic field therapy (NCCAM, 2013).

The 2007 National Health Interview Survey indicates that 38% of adults and 12% of children had used CAM (Ventola, 2010). CAM is often used in conjunction with other diagnostic, treatment, or prevention strategies. Families who have had a negative experience with conventional medicine may choose alternative or complementary therapies, particularly for children with chronic illnesses. The pediatric healthcare provider should know what therapies patients and families are using, have basic working knowledge of such treatments, and be able to offer information to support the families' use of CAM therapies for their children. The nurse or APRN should also assess whether the family has employed cultural practices, ethnic routines, or religious rituals that might include the use of herbs, medicines, or the wearing of certain charms.

Education

In a 2014 position statement, the Society of Pediatric Nurses (SPN) outlined education guidelines for the registered nurse level of pediatric nursing with the intent to prepare prelicensure students and new graduates for the complex care of children and their families (SPN, 2014). The position statement contains five recommendations that address required curricula, theoretical and clinical content, and qualifications of pediatric faculty. The overarching concept in this position statement is that educational programs must contain content related to patient- and family-centered care in a "freestanding" pediatric nursing course. SPN states that critical issues have affected current health care and create challenges in educating pediatric nurses. This document serves as a guiding force to direct nursing education for the care of children in a complex society. Pediatric nurses, in collaboration with nursing faculty, help to provide key learning and clinical experiences for students.

Prelicensure education for the registered nurse may occur in a variety of programs, including baccalaureate and graduate entry programs, associate degree programs, or perhaps a hospital diploma program. In 1986, the American Association of Colleges of Nursing (AACN) published *The Essentials of Baccalaureate Education for Professional Nursing Practice*, a landmark set of core educational standards for the professional nurse. The most current edition (2008) continues to provide direction for the education of professional nurses in the 21st century. *Essentials* defines the professional nurse as "that individual prepared with a minimum of a baccalaureate in nursing but is also inclusive of one who *enters* professional practice with a master's degree in nursing or a nursing doctorate" (AACN, 2008, p. 38).

Educational content regarding genomics and genetics has also been incorporated into nursing curricula. *Essential Nursing Competencies and Curricula Guidelines for Genetics and Genomics*, written by the Consensus Panel on Genetic/Genomic Competencies (2008), with outcome indicators established by consensus in 2008, outlines the role of the nurse in applying and integrating genetic and genomic knowledge in the processes of screening, assessment, referral, and provision of education, care, and support. Numerous nursing organizations, including the AAN, ANA, the National League for Nursing, NAPNAP, NONPF, and SPN, have endorsed this document.

Post-baccalaureate education for the pediatric advanced practice registered nurse is required at the master's or doctoral level. In 1996, with updates in 2008 and 2011, the AACN published *The Essentials of Master's Education for Advanced Practice Nursing*. This document outlines generic core curriculum content for all advanced practice nursing students, including research, policy, organization, financing of health care, ethics, professional role development, theoretical foundations of nursing practice, human diversity and social issues, and health promotion and disease prevention. A specialty core curriculum for APRNs who provide direct clinical care includes advanced health and physical assessment, advanced pathophysiology, advanced pharmacology, and additional clinical experiences.

The National Association of Clinical Nurse Specialists (NACNS) developed a *Statement on CNS Practice and Education* that provides a framework for a first level assessment of core CNS competencies regardless of specialty (NACNS, 2010). Similarly, the National Organization of Nurse Practitioner Faculties (NONPF) has developed curriculum guidelines for nurse practitioners, incorporating the full scope of advanced nursing practice (NONPF, 2013). These guidelines and standards apply to graduate education and emphasize direct care across settings. The education of the pediatric advanced practice registered nurse includes specialty content in advanced health and physical assessment of the child, advanced physiology and pathophysiology, pediatric pharmacology, advanced child and family development, family theory, promotion and maintenance of optimal health for children and families, and management of acute and chronic conditions in children.

Clinical practicum experiences for CNS and PNP students in a variety of settings are a vital part of the advanced practice curriculum. Clinical experience builds on course work and simulation and is designed to enable graduates to collect health data, establish a diagnosis, identify expected outcomes individualized to the child and family, plan and prescribe care, implement interventions, and evaluate the child's and family's progress toward attainment of outcomes. In clinical settings, students are expected to provide high-level nursing care based on current clinical evidence and guidelines that incorporate technical skill, critical thinking, leadership, theoretical knowledge, and clinical scholarship. Academic faculty responsible for the overall implementation of advanced practice programs are ideally prepared at the doctoral level and are actively engaged in practice settings with children and families as clinicians, educators, or researchers. Preceptors with outstanding clinical expertise actively collaborate with educators and students to guide clinical education. In some academic institutions, preceptors may qualify for courtesy or clinical faculty appointments.

In the past decade, nurse leaders and educators examined educational programs that prepare advanced practice registered nurses and reviewed reports and projections for healthcare needs of the 21st century. It was evident that the educational preparation and provision of services by advanced practice registered nurses, coupled with the complexity of health care in the United States, demanded a transformation. The American Association of Colleges of

Nursing (AACN) recommended that the future education of advanced practice registered nurses (clinical nurse specialists and nurse practitioners) would occur at the doctoral level as a Doctor of Nursing Practice (DNP). AACN recommended that this shift to doctoral preparation should occur by 2015. Additionally, many nurses have and will continue to earn doctorate degrees in philosophy, nursing science, and education. These nurses are prepared for a wide range of practice environments and responsibilities, including advanced roles in academia, education, and research.

In preparing for this transition in education, the AACN charged a committee to develop *The Essentials of Doctoral Education for Advanced Nursing Practice* (AACN, 2006). This document incorporates and expands on the *Master's Essentials*, currently used to guide advanced practice registered nurse education, to ensure the necessary academic and clinical rigor required for DNP education. The eight essentials for doctoral education include:

I. Scientific underpinnings for practice

II. Organizational and systems leadership for quality improvement and systems thinking

III. Clinical scholarship and analytical methods for evidence-based practice

IV. Information systems and technology, and patient care technology, for the improvement and transformation of health care

V. Healthcare policy for advocacy in health care

VI. Interprofessional collaboration for improving patient and population health outcomes

VII. Clinical prevention and population health for improving the nation's health

VIII. Advanced nursing practice

Additional work has been done to guide faculty in developing curricula and to set accreditation standards for programs. Advanced practice nursing education will now align with audiology, medicine, pharmacy, and physical therapy in preparing practitioners with a terminal, doctoral-level practice degree.

Certification

Certification is a process by which an independent, nongovernmental agency recognizes an individual nurse's qualifications and knowledge for specialty nursing practice. All pediatric nurses should obtain certification. The nurse achieves specialty certification credentials through the completion of specialized education, experience in specialty nursing practice, and the successful completion of a qualifying examination. Maintenance of certification is accomplished through a variety of mechanisms including reexamination, continuing education, self-assessment, and ongoing clinical practice. Through this process, the agency or professional organization acknowledges to the individual and the general public that the nurse has mastered a body of knowledge for a particular specialty. Certification is evolving, with multiple opportunities for certification available (Table 3). The nurse should be informed about which certification option is appropriate for him or her.

Regulation

State jurisdictions have regulatory and legal oversight of practice for the RN and APRN. Considerable variability exists between states in the implementation of this oversight, and APRN statutes vary widely from title protection to a more specific delineation of APRN practice. The autonomy of practice varies as well, ranging from private and independent practice with the ability to refer patients to other healthcare providers to physician-supervised practice. In 2008, the APRN Consensus Work Group and the National Council of State Boards of Nursing APRN Advisory Committee produced a *Consensus Model for APRN Regulation: Licensure, Accreditation, Certification and Education.* The model defined the roles of APRN practice as Certified Nurse Practitioner (CNP), Certified Registered Nurse Anesthetist (CRNA), Certified Nurse Midwife (CNM), and Clinical Nurse Specialist (CNS). It recommended national standardization of scope of practice based on population foci, licensure, and education received from a nationally accredited program that ensured educational requirements. It also recommended that APRN certification programs be accredited by a national certification accrediting body and require a continued competency mechanism. The model is intended to be fully implemented by 2015 (APRN, 2008).

ANA supports one scope of nursing practice, one licensure for registered nurses, and minimal statutory language about advanced practice registered nurses. ANA also proposes that state boards of nursing promote specific designations of APRN roles in rules and regulations instead of law to avoid attaching statutory language to the roles. Additionally, the profession should self-regulate RN and APRN roles through consistent standards of practice, certification, peer review, and continuing education to retain the responsibility and accountability for such regulation.

TABLE 3. Pediatric Nursing Certification Opportunities

Certifying Organization	Certification Available
American Nurses Credentialing Center (ANCC)	Child/Adolescent Psychiatric and Mental Health Clinical Nurse Specialist (PMHCNS-BC)* last testing in 2016* with recertification only Pediatric Clinical Nurse Specialist (PCNS-BC)* last testing in 2017* Recertification will still be available. Pediatric Nurse (RN-BC) Pediatric Primary Care Nurse Practitioner (PPCNP-BC) School Nurse Practitioner (SNP-BC)*
American Association of Critical Care Nurses: AACN Certification Corporation	Critical Care Registered Nurse – Pediatric (CCRN-P) Critical Care Registered Nurse – Neonatal (CCRN-N) Pediatric Clinical Nurse Specialist (ACCNS-P) – Wellness through acute care (pediatric) Neonatal Clinical Nurse Specialist (ACCNS-N) – Wellness through acute care (neonatal)
Oncology Nursing Certification Corporation	Certified Pediatric Hematology Oncology Nurse (CPHON)
National Board for Certification of School Nurses (NBCSN)	Nationally Certified School Nurse (NCSN)
Hospice & Palliative Care Credentialing Center (HPCC)	Certified Hospice and Palliative Pediatric Nurse (CHPPN)
National Certification Corporation (NCC)	Low-risk Neonatal Nurse (RNC) Neonatal Intensive Care Nurse (RNC) Neonatal Nurse Practitioner (NNP)
Pediatric Nursing Certification Board (PNCB)	Certified Pediatric Nurse Practitioner – Primary Care (CPNP-PC) Certified Pediatric Nurse Practitioner – Acute Care (CPNP-AC) Certified Pediatric Nurse (CPN) Certified Pediatric Emergency Nurse (CPEN) Pediatric Primary Care Mental Health Specialist (PMHS)

* Certification is no longer offered but able to be maintained

Ethical Issues in Pediatric Care

Pediatric care is delivered in an environment of specialized knowledge and skill under circumstances in which opportunities for ethical deliberation and reflection may be less than ideal. Parents and families are emotionally stressed and, in some instances, they themselves may be patients. Staffing and other organizational issues may introduce additional stress on the care team. These examples only emphasize the importance of viewing the pediatric care unit as a moral community in which ethical reflection, discussion, and action are as much a part of a care plan as diagnosis and treatment. Viewing ethics in this context also allows for an understanding of ethical issues that are both broad and deep, encompassing ethical distress that may occur within oneself, among members of the care team, and between the care team and families.

ANA states that "respect for the inherent worth, dignity, and human rights of every individual is a fundamental principle that underlies all nursing practice" (ANA, 2010). Each individual nurse has accepted the ethical obligations of the profession in addition to the individual capacity to make moral choices as human beings. While this provides a rich legacy, it can also be a source of ethical uncertainty or conflict. Nurses should consult their state board of nursing, institutional policies, and professional code of ethics in situations of ethical distress. In some cases, a healthy professional distance allows nurses to carry out decisions that are ethically permissible, although not the choices nurses would make for their own children.

How pediatric nurses understand what constitutes an ethical dilemma can influence their ability to identify ethical issues, discuss them with colleagues, and take action to resolve or ameliorate ethical conflict. Understanding the unit as a moral community includes not only how nurses treat patients, but also how nurses treat each other. Differences in cultural or religious backgrounds, hierarchy, or power, which are often unspoken but powerful influences, can enrich or impede how a unit functions. All members of the healthcare team must have a realistic understanding of ethics as an everyday concern rather than an issue of crisis management. This creates an environment in which high standards are the rule rather than the exception, providing support for a community characterized by mutual respect and willingness to take responsibility for lapses and improvements. ANA's *Code of Ethics for Nurses with Interpretive Statements* (ANA, 2015) makes explicit the primary goals, values, and obligations of the profession of nursing to patients, families, and each other.

This code of ethics provides principles based on important moral values that shape the nurse's professional identity and provides the nurse with the foundation to apply the principles in his or her work setting. Although there is a tendency to put difficult cases behind oneself as quickly as possible and move on, ethical growth requires that nurses reflect on their practice to identify and reinforce what was done well and learn from inexperience and mistakes. Nursing codes of ethics provide principles based on important moral values that shape the nurse's professional identity (Butts & Rich, 2013) and provide the nurse with the foundation to apply the principles in his or her work setting.

The nine provisions included in ANA's *Code of Ethics for Nurses with Interpretive Statements* (2015) are listed below with examples that are relevant to pediatric nursing.

Provision 1. The nurse practices with compassion and respect for the inherent dignity, worth, and unique attributes of every person.

Occasionally, a case presents itself that challenges the professional relationship between the caregiver and the patient/family. In one situation, a nurse assumed care for a young black male child who was not diagnosed right away when he came in for multiple pneumonias and respiratory issues. The family was devastated when the child was diagnosed with cystic fibrosis, rare in black males. The nurse took care of the child and his family every time the child was admitted to the hospital and felt that no one could take care of the child as well as she could. The family and nurse became very close and the nurse even made home visits. The parents relied on the nurse for moral support as well as for the care of the child. The nurse became very angry and protective when the child lost his developmental milestones due to a brain infection. Fortunately, an empathetic colleague pulled her aside one day and said, "You cannot take care of him today, I will. You must start to set boundaries and pull yourself away a little bit." To set boundaries is hard. Ethically, the nurse was not the parent or caretaker and had crossed the line between compassion and respect for a nonprofessional relationship.

Provision 2. The nurse's primary commitment is to the patient, whether an individual, family, group, community, or population.

When parents insist on prolonged life-supporting therapy and the provider teams allow it, such action can challenge both a nurse's professional identity and personal moral agency. How a nurse handles such situations is as ethically important as the course of action he or she chooses to take. Pediatric nurses who provide care for infants and children born with congenital defects can encounter a variety of situations that provide an ethical challenge. Healthcare providers diagnose complex congenital conditions in a fetus as young as 15 weeks gestation, giving rise to ethical questions of pregnancy termination, intrauterine surgical intervention risking fetal demise, and post-delivery care.

One case of this difficult decision-making was encountered in the first fetal ultrasound done after a confirmed pregnancy in a couple who had multiple attempts at in vitro fertilization. The ultrasound revealed complex congenital heart disease that would require open-heart surgery within the first week of the baby's life. The couple decided to continue the pregnancy and plan for delivery of a term baby—if the pregnancy could be maintained until term. Delivery and neonatal cardiac surgery would occur at a hospital in another state away from supportive family and friends.

The baby survived the initial surgery but required many more procedures and interventions. After several months in the hospital, the baby could not be weaned off a ventilator and required peritoneal dialysis for renal function and intravenous inotropes to maintain cardiac output. While providing excellent intensive care for the baby, the pediatric nurses continued to support the baby's parents even though the prognosis was grim. After an ethics consult and with support from the palliative care, medical, and surgical teams, the pediatric nurses supported the grieving parents when they realized their baby would not survive to enjoy the quality of life they desired. End-of-life options were discussed and eventually the baby was extubated while being held by his parents.

Provision 3. The nurse promotes, advocates for, and strives to protect the rights, health, and safety of the patient.

Children spend a large portion of their day attending school. The school nurse is often aware of health and social issues for the children in his or her care and has the responsibility to advocate on their behalf. In one case, a 7-year-old child with asthma had been in the school nurse's office almost every day for two weeks with complaints of difficulty breathing. The child did not have access to medication at school, despite the nurse's frequent calls to the family to inquire about an inhaler. Eventually, the nurse learned from the child that he and his family were living with friends because they were evicted from their apartment. The friends were smokers and had several cats.

The child did not have health insurance to acquire the needed asthma medication. Through many phone calls and inquiries, the school nurse linked the family with social services to provide the necessary health insurance and a better living environment. She also collaborated with the primary care provider to evaluate and treat the child's asthma. The nurse provided asthma education for the family and child and evaluated the child's response to the newly acquired asthma prescriptions. She provided ongoing assessments to assure continued care for the child. Through the advocacy efforts of the school nurse, the child received the health care he needed to control his asthma.

Provision 4. The nurse has authority, accountability, and responsibility for nursing practice; makes decisions; and takes action consistent with the obligation to promote health and provide optimal care.

The nursing care structure of a general surgical pediatric unit includes registered nurses (RNs) who work with certified nursing assistants (CNAs) to provide care for a group of six to eight patients. The CNA is traditionally responsible for obtaining vital signs, assisting with bathing, providing nutrition, turning and positioning as needed, and other designated tasks. A child was admitted to a general surgical pediatric unit following a nephrectomy for a Wilms' tumor. The child had some hemodynamic instability during the surgical procedure, but was stabilized leaving the post-anesthesia care unit (PACU). The RN personally evaluated the patient and took his vital signs upon his admission to the pediatric floor. She determined that, because of the instability during surgery, the child would require continued close monitoring, so, to provide optimum patient care, she chose to monitor the patient herself as opposed to directing the CNA to take the vital signs.

Provision 5. The nurse owes the same duties to self as to others, including the responsibility to promote health and safety, preserve wholeness of character and integrity, maintain competence, and continue personal and professional growth.

The nursing staff on an inpatient pediatric hematology/oncology/bone marrow transplant unit in a children's hospital received a significant gift from the family of one of their patients to provide a scholarship for nursing education. The family designated the gift for this unit in thanks for exceptional care their child received over multiple admissions and many years, including a bone marrow transplant. The unit-based nursing committee, with concurrence from the donors, felt they should use this gift to support the education of many nurses instead of just one or two.

Based upon the committee decision and the lack of any local nursing (or interprofessional) conferences specific to the care of the pediatric hematology/oncology/bone marrow transplant population, two of the unit nurses on this committee volunteered to organize a local conference directed at the care of this specific population.

These two nurses planned a one-day conference comprised of local, regional, and international speakers who presented content on new medical treatments, end-of-life care, and psychosocial interventions. The conference was marketed to all nurses and members of interprofessional care teams in the local and regional area who cared for or were interested in pediatric patients with cancer and blood disorders. More than 100 healthcare professionals attended the conference. Continuing education units were provided to enable specialty certification for conference attendees.

Provision 6. The nurse, through individual and collective effort, establishes, maintains, and improves the ethical environment of the work setting and conditions of employment that are conducive to safe, quality health care.

Many institutions promote employee participation in shared governance as a concept in nursing care delivery. However, a lack of practical application can be problematic. The pediatric nurse who focuses on providing patient- and family-centered care and applying current research evidence in practice requires reasonable work hours and resources. Pediatric nurses and advanced practice registered nurses are responsible for advocating for equitable work, sick leave, and vacation leave schedules that do not require them to neglect either personal or professional priorities. The pediatric population, whose organs are still developing, can be easily susceptible to communicable diseases. If nurses get sick, they cannot deliver the quality care that their patients deserve and may even place their patients in jeopardy.

In one situation, a nurse was working in a busy pediatric unit that was short-staffed. For a few days, she had felt the early symptoms of a cold and her symptoms were getting worse. The nurse was concerned about leaving her coworkers short, but rather than jeopardizing the health of the patients, chose to obtain her supervisor's permission to remove herself from the floor. These types of initiatives taken on a regular basis promote health and well-being both for the nurses and the families and children they serve.

Provision 7. The nurse, in all roles and settings, advances the profession through research and scholarly inquiry, professional standards development, and the generation of both nursing and health policy.

The nurse manager of a large pediatric intensive care unit recognized that several patients with complex medical issues were discharged but had to return within a short time period. Many of these children were readmitted because of a lack of family knowledge and experience in performing ordered therapies. The manager realized that changes in staff management of the children prior to discharge were necessary for their successful transfer back to family care. She engaged a small group of the nursing staff to evaluate the process of transfer and discharge and found some disconnects in the system. The manager worked with nursing administration and representatives from the PICU and pediatric units to complete a quality improvement project that identified the need for collaborative discharge planning and parental education. Through this project, the nurse manager trained the interprofessional team on how to educate parents to care for their child's condition and coordinated planning for close follow up of the children after they went home. Her successful improvement program and staff training cut back on the frequency of the children's readmittance, allowing their parents to care for them at home.

Provision 8. The nurse collaborates with other health professionals and the public to protect human rights, promote health diplomacy, and reduce health disparities.

Pediatric registered nurses and advanced practice registered nurses collaborate with many members of the healthcare team daily. At each intersection of the healthcare experience—including primary care, school, emergency departments, urgent care facilities, and after-school or sports programs—pediatric nurses maintain strong and effective communication with all members of the healthcare team to meet the needs of children. Pediatric registered nurses and advanced practice registered nurses often advance legislation to protect the health and well-being of children. Examples include car seat safety and all-terrain vehicle legislation shepherded through the legislative process often by pediatric nurses and APRNs.

Pediatric registered nurses and advanced practice registered nurses volunteer across the world in response to natural and man-made disasters and in areas where children are at a clear disadvantage. Pediatric nurses and APRNs participate in medical missionary trips and answer calls for emergency pediatric care and support. They are a vital link to children receiving critical services including life-saving or life-changing medical treatment, emergency disaster care, and health and nutrition information and education. Their reach can be felt from their local communities to countries across the globe in need.

Provision 9. The profession of nursing, collectively through its professional organizations, must articulate nursing values, maintain the integrity of the profession, and integrate principles of social justice into nursing and health policy.

Many pediatric nurses and advanced practice registered nurses belong to professional associations, which may be broadly defined by population (e.g., pediatrics) or pediatric sub-specialty. Through their associations, RNs and APRNs can shape social policy by participating in local member events, letter-writing campaigns to local and national legislators, and leadership development opportunities. These organizations articulate nursing values through professional journal publications and may provide information and materials such as advocacy tool kits to help their members speak out on issues important to the profession and to the children and families they serve.

Pediatric state and national organizations hold legislative days in Washington, DC, or their state capital where pediatric nurses, advanced practice registered nurses, and undergraduate and graduate nursing students meet with congressional representatives to advocate for the nursing profession and the nation's children. An example of how this has been effective is through the efforts of APRNs to change social policy and legislation in 19 states where full practice authority has been granted to nurse practitioners.

Advocacy in Pediatric Care

Every pediatric nurse is a child advocate. Advocacy occurs in practice settings, committee meetings, agency discussions, public settings, and parent meetings, sometimes on a daily basis. Advocacy means providing a voice for those unheard, ensuring that important issues are addressed (Putman, 2014). Pediatric nurses have many essential advocacy qualities: strong communication skills, negotiation, awareness of patient needs, perseverance, leadership, people skills, and the ability to both multitask and think innovatively "outside the workplace." Because of their specialized knowledge, holistic approach, and understanding of the context of child health, pediatric nurses are uniquely qualified to assist in the creation, implementation, and evaluation of policies at all levels. Pediatric nurses can advocate by finding passion related to their work, community, or personal interests. Examples of advocacy opportunities include learning about important local and national issues, joining workplace and professional association committees, getting involved in community activities, and writing letters to local and national representatives.

Pediatric nurses understand both child and family needs, placing them in a prime position to advocate for those identified needs. Because of their expertise, pediatric nurses can see the effects of policy decisions on the health and well-being of patients and families. Professional values, such as possessing an ethical framework, abiding by the *Code of Ethics for Nurses with Interpretive Statements* (ANA, 2015), and acknowledging the mission and goals of professional organizations, can guide the nurse in advocacy efforts. Nurses have demonstrated advocacy success in areas surrounding the development of safe playgrounds, choking prevention, ensuring healthier school lunch programs, and assuring funding and services in state children's health insurance programs (SCHIP).

Continued Commitment to the Profession

Pediatric nurses are committed to:

- Demonstrating excellent nursing practice consistent with professional nursing standards, specialty nursing standards, and state boards of registered nursing regulations for registered nurses and advanced practice registered nurses.

- Supporting education and role development of novice practitioners by serving as preceptors, role models, and mentors.

- Advancing the profession through enhancing public awareness and community activities.

- Maintaining active membership in professional organizations.

- Working to influence policy-making bodies to improve access to quality health care.

- Using an ethical framework to evaluate issues regarding care.

- Demonstrating practice consistent with ethical and legal standards in compliance with state and federal regulations.

- Developing and implementing evidence-based guidelines.

- The scholarship of discovery through conducting and participating in research.

Furthermore, pediatric nurses are committed to working together to address common issues regardless of practice roles, settings, or professional affiliations. In so doing, they merge their knowledge, insights, resources, and goals, strengthening health care for the children and families to whom they are ultimately accountable.

Standards of Pediatric Nursing Practice

Standards of Practice

Standard 1. Assessment
The pediatric registered nurse collects comprehensive data pertinent to the child's health and/or the situation.

Competencies
The pediatric registered nurse:

- Collects data in a systematic and ongoing process that conveys respect for the child and family.

- Involves the child, family, other individuals important to the family, and other healthcare providers, as appropriate, in holistic data collection.

- Elicits the values, preferences, expressed needs, and knowledge of the child and family related to the healthcare situation.

- Utilizes the preferred language of the family through a culturally sensitive process and seeks a qualified interpreter if necessary.

- Assesses the child's and family's environment for facilitators and barriers to growth and development (e.g., environmental toxins, safe play areas).

- Prioritizes data collection activities based on the child's immediate condition, situation, and anticipated needs.

- Uses analytical models and problem-solving tools to collect data systematically.

- Interprets available data, information, and knowledge relevant to the situation to identify and document patterns and variances.

- Obtains data from information systems to include complete and appropriate information.

- Documents relevant data in a retrievable form.

- Bases assessment techniques on research and knowledge, using clinical judgment to ensure that relevant and necessary data is collected.

- Synthesizes available data, information, and knowledge relevant to the situation to identify patterns and variances.

- Uses appropriate evidence-based assessment techniques specific for the child's age in collecting pertinent data.

- In addition to basic history and physical skills expected for every age group, pediatric nursing assessment of infants, children, and adolescents should include the following foci (a comprehensive list can be found in Appendix A):

  — Measurement of child's length/height, weight, and body mass index with comparison to age-specific percentiles. It is particularly important to consider prenatal and perinatal history and postnatal course in all foci.

  — Developmental assessment, including physical, motor, social, and cognitive development with reference to age-appropriate tasks and sequence. Tools are available to assist nurses with consistent evaluation and measurement of developmental progress or deficits.

  — Behavioral assessment with reference to history and expected behaviors for age. Examples are children with learning- or school-related problems such as attention deficit, hyperactivity, or oppositional defiant disorders.

  — Family composition and function with reference to patterns of interaction, parenting style and discipline practices, and principles of anticipatory guidance.

  — Recognition of developmental delays, genetic disorders, child abuse, and neglect; assessment of pubertal changes and the need for reproductive education in adolescents, stemming from appropriate assessment, intervention, and referral.

Additional competencies for the advanced practice registered nurse

The advanced practice registered nurse:

- Collaborates with other professionals to assemble a comprehensive assessment of the child and family.

- Conducts comprehensive physical, mental health, and developmental assessments.

- Analyzes the family system to identify factors that might influence the health of the child and family.

- Screens for evidence-based risk factors (e.g., unsupervised after school, abuse, bullying, and relationships with peers and siblings).

- Initiates and interprets age-appropriate and condition-specific laboratory tests and diagnostic procedures.

- Assesses the quality of care provided to children and families across settings.

Standard 2. Diagnosis

The pediatric registered nurse analyzes the assessment data to determine diagnoses or issues.

Competencies

The pediatric registered nurse:

- Derives diagnoses appropriate to their scope of practice or issues based on assessment data that are developmentally appropriate and specific to areas of growth and development, age, cultural sensitivity, and family dynamics.

- Validates diagnoses or issues with the child, family, significant others, and other healthcare providers when possible and appropriate.

- Identifies actual or potential risks to the child's health and safety or barriers to health, which may include but are not limited to interpersonal, systematic, or environmental circumstances.

- Uses standardized classification systems and clinical decision support tools, when available, in identifying diagnoses.

- Documents diagnoses or issues in a manner that facilitates the determination of expected outcomes and plan of care.

Additional competencies for the advanced practice registered nurse

The advanced practice registered nurse:

- Systematically compares and contrasts clinical findings with normal and abnormal variations and developmental events in formulating a differential diagnosis that encompasses anatomical, physiological, motor, cognitive, developmental, psychological, and social behavior across the pediatric lifespan.

- Utilizes complex data and information obtained during interview, examination, and diagnostic procedures in identifying diagnoses.

- Assists staff in developing and maintaining competency in the diagnostic process.

- Interprets age-, developmental-, and situational-appropriate screening and analytic studies essential in the diagnosis and management of the child with a health condition.

- Applies evidence-based clinical practice guidelines to guide screening and diagnosis.

Standard 3. Outcomes Identification

The pediatric registered nurse identifies expected outcomes for a plan individualized to the child, family, or situation.

Competencies

The pediatric registered nurse:

- Involves the child, family, and other healthcare providers in formulating expected outcomes when possible and appropriate.

- Develops expected outcomes from the diagnosis that are developmentally appropriate, age-specific, family-centered, and culturally and spiritually sensitive.

- Develops expected outcomes that are realistic in relation to the child and family's potential capabilities and available resources.

- Formulates and defines expected outcomes considering the child's condition, the child's and family's expectations, associated risks, benefits, costs, current scientific evidence, and the nurse's clinical expertise.

- Includes a realistic timeframe for attainment of expected outcomes.

- Develops expected outcomes that ensure continuity of care.

- Identifies expected outcomes that consider the implementation of evidence-based practices.

- Modifies expected outcomes based on changes in the status of the child and family and emergence of external changes.

- Documents expected outcomes that are measurable and attainable.

Additional competencies for the advanced practice registered nurse

The advanced practice registered nurse:

- Identifies expected outcomes that incorporate cost and clinical effectiveness, the child's and family's expectations, and continuity and consistency among healthcare providers.

- Differentiates outcomes that require care process interventions from those that require system-level interventions.

- Incorporates the use of evidence-based clinical guidelines that support positive expected outcomes for the child.

Standard 4. Planning

The pediatric registered nurse develops a plan that prescribes strategies and alternatives to attain expected outcomes.

Competencies

The pediatric registered nurse:

- Develops an individualized plan of care considering the child's characteristics and the situation, including age, growth, developmental level, values, beliefs, spiritual and health practices, choices, coping style, cultural and environmental factors, and available technology.

- Develops the plan of care in conjunction with the child (when developmentally able), family, and others, as appropriate.

- Formulates a plan of care that is family-centered, reflects current pediatric nursing practice, and takes into consideration the family's cultural, spiritual, and health practice needs; ability to read and write; level of health literacy; and capacity for understanding complex healthcare processes.

- Includes strategies within the plan of care that address each identified diagnosis or issue, such as promotion and restoration of health; prevention of illness, injury, and disease; alleviation of suffering; and supportive end-of-life care.

- Includes strategies for health, wholeness, and wellness across the lifespan.

- Includes synthesis of the family's values and beliefs regarding nursing and medical therapies within the plan of care.

- Provides for continuity within the plan of care.

- Provides for special confidentiality and privacy needs when necessary.

- Incorporates an implementation pathway or timeline within the plan of care that is dynamic, flexible, and reassessed at established intervals and as needed.

- Reevaluates the plan of care with the child, family, and others, as appropriate.

- Utilizes the plan of care to provide direction to other members of the healthcare team.

- Defines the plan of care to reflect current statutes, rules and regulations, and standards.

- Integrates current trends, scientific evidence, and research affecting care into the planning process.

- Explores practice settings, safe spaces, and time for the nurse, child, and other healthcare providers to investigate suggested, potential, and alternative options.

- Considers the economic impact of the plan of care.

- Documents the plan of care using standardized language or recognized terminology.

- Confirms that the comprehensive plan of care includes educational interventions related to the child's health status, conventional and alternative therapies, self-care activities, appropriate referrals, and coordination of comprehensive services to ensure continuity of care.

Additional competencies for the advanced practice registered nurse

The advanced practice registered nurse:

- Identifies assessment, diagnostic strategies, and therapeutic interventions within the plan of care that reflect current pediatric healthcare practice, including data, research, literature, and expert clinical knowledge.

- Devises a comprehensive plan of care that reflects the responsibilities of the advanced practice registered nurse, child, and family and may include delegation of activities.

- Leads the design and development of interprofessional processes to address the situation or issue.

- Formulates the comprehensive plan of care, including educational interventions related to the child's health status, conventional and alternative therapies, self-care activities, and coordination of comprehensive services to ensure continuity of care.

- Identifies the need for and initiates appropriate referrals to healthcare professionals to support the comprehensive plan of care.

- Documents the comprehensive plan of care in a manner that allows access by the child, family, and healthcare providers, as appropriate, and provides direction for the family and healthcare team as they focus on attaining expected outcomes.

- Selects or designs strategies to meet the multifaceted needs of the complex pediatric patient.

- Contributes to the development and continuous improvement of organizational systems that support the plan of care process.

- Supports the integration of clinical, human, and financial resources to enhance and complete the decision-making processes.

Standard 5. Implementation

The pediatric registered nurse implements the identified plan.

Competencies

The pediatric registered nurse:

- Partners with the child, family, and other caregivers, as appropriate, to implement the plan in a safe, realistic, and timely manner.

- Encourages the child of accountable age and ability to assume responsibility related to his or her care.

- Provides holistic care that addresses the needs of diverse pediatric populations.

- Demonstrates caring behaviors towards children and families.

- Utilizes technology to measure, record, and retrieve healthcare data, implement the nursing process, and enhance pediatric nursing practice.

- Counsels the child and family in resolving issues or making determinations of what the next appropriate steps might be.

- Implements the plan of care in a safe, cost-effective, and timely manner.

- Documents implementation and any modifications, including changes or omissions, of the identified plan of care.

- Utilizes evidence-based interventions and treatments specific to the diagnosis or problem.

- Utilizes community resources and systems to implement the plan of care and coordinates access to appropriate resources.

- Collaborates with nursing colleagues and others to implement the plan of care.

- Advocates for health care that is timely and sensitive to the needs of pediatric patients, with particular emphasis on the needs of diverse populations.

- Applies appropriate knowledge of major health problems as well as knowledge of cultural diversity in implementing the plan of care.

- Accommodates different styles of communication with the child and family.

- Integrates traditional and complementary healthcare practices as appropriate.
- Documents the implementation of and any modifications, changes, or omissions to the plan of care.

Additional competencies for the advanced practice registered nurse

The advanced practice registered nurse:

- Facilitates utilization of systems and community resources to implement the plan of care.
- Supports collaboration with nursing and other colleagues to implement the plan.
- Incorporates new knowledge and strategies to initiate change in nursing care practices if desired outcomes are not achieved.
- Assumes responsibility for safe and efficient implementation of the plan.
- Uses advanced communication skills to promote relationships between the child, family, and caregiver to assure an open discussion of the family's experiences and to improve healthcare outcomes.
- Actively participates in the development and continuous improvement of systems that support implementation of the plan.

Standard 5A. Coordination of Care

The pediatric registered nurse coordinates care delivery.

Competencies

The pediatric registered nurse:

- Organizes components of the plan of care.

- Documents coordination of the care.

- Provides education to the child, family, and caregiver that includes health promotion, anticipatory guidance, information about injury and disease prevention, and home care management as appropriate for the child's developmental level.

- Manages a child's care in order to maximize independence and quality of life.

- Assists the child and family to identify options for alternative care.

- Provides consistent communication during transitions in care.

- Advocates for the delivery of dignified and humane care by the interprofessional team.

- Identifies and coordinates access to appropriate community resources.

Additional competencies for the advanced practice registered nurse

The advanced practice registered nurse:

- Provides leadership in the coordination of interprofessional health care for integrated delivery of pediatric care services.

- Synthesizes data and information to prescribe necessary system and community support measures, including modifications of surroundings.

- Delegates appropriate activities according to the condition of the child and the relative skill and scope of practice of the caregiver.

- Provides case management and clinical coordination of care using advanced data synthesis with consideration of the child's and family's complex needs and desired outcomes.

- Coordinates system and community resources to achieve optimal quality of care, delivered in a cost-effective manner within an inter-professional team approach.

- Negotiates health-related services and additional specialized care with the child, family, appropriate systems, agencies, and providers across continuums of care.

- Discusses referrals with the child (if age appropriate) and family.

- Makes referrals to other healthcare providers and community service agencies as appropriate to meet the needs of the child with consideration of benefits and costs.

- Ensures continuity of care throughout the healthcare referral process by implementing recommendations from referral sources.

Standard 5B. Health Teaching and Health Promotion

The pediatric registered nurse employs strategies to promote health and a safe environment.

Competencies

The pediatric registered nurse:

- Provides health teaching, based on current scientific knowledge, research, epidemiological principles, and the family's health beliefs and practices, that addresses such topics as healthy lifestyles, risk-reducing behaviors, developmental needs, daily activities, and preventive self-care.

- Uses health promotion and health teaching methods appropriate to the situation and to the child's and family's developmental levels, learning needs, readiness, ability to learn, language preference, and culture.

- Provides information on the risks and benefits, intended effects, and potential adverse effects of proposed therapies and healthcare practices.

- Seeks opportunities for feedback and evaluation of the strategies' effectiveness.

- Utilizes technology to design and communicate health information and pediatric education appropriate to the child's culture, age, developmental and cognitive levels, and readiness and ability to learn.

- Evaluates health information resources within the area of practice, such as the Internet, for accuracy, readability, and comprehensibility to help the child and family access quality health information.

Additional competencies for the advanced practice registered nurse

The advanced practice registered nurse:

- Employs diverse and complex strategies, interventions, and teaching with the child and family to promote, maintain, restore, and improve health and to prevent illness and injury.

- Synthesizes empirical evidence about risk behaviors, learning theories, behavioral change theories, motivational theories, epidemiology, genetics, culture, and other related theories and frameworks when designing health education information and programs.

- Bases anticipatory guidance and teaching on current scientific knowledge, research, epidemiological principles, and the family's health beliefs and practices.

- Collaborates with the interprofessional team to provide the child (if age appropriate) and family with information regarding interventions, including potential benefits, risks, complications, and alternatives.

- Engages consumer alliances and advocacy groups, when appropriate, in health teaching and health promotion activities related to the health and welfare of children and families.

Standard 5C. Consultation

The advanced practice registered nurse provides consultation to influence the identified plan of care for children, enhance the abilities of others, and effect change in the healthcare system.

Competencies

The advanced practice registered nurse:

- Synthesizes data, information, theoretical frameworks, and evidence when providing consultation.

- Bases consultation on mutual respect among the child, family, and other primary caregivers.

- Facilitates the effectiveness of a consultation by involving the stakeholders in the decision-making process.

- Communicates consultation recommendations that influence the identified plan of care, facilitate understanding by involved stakeholders, enhance the work of others, and effect change.

- Initiates and provides appropriate consultation to implement the interprofessional plan of care for the child with consideration given to the child's unique developmental needs and aptitudes and the family's level of adaptation and ability to cope with the child's health concerns.

Standard 5D. Prescriptive Authority and Treatment

The advanced practice registered nurse uses prescriptive authority, procedures, referrals, treatments, and therapies in accordance with state and federal laws and regulations.

Competencies

The advanced practice registered nurse:

- Prescribes evidence-based treatments, therapies, and procedures considering the child's comprehensive healthcare needs and based on current pediatric knowledge, research, and practice.

- Prescribes appropriate non-pharmacological interventions, including complementary and alternative therapies.

- Prescribes pharmacologic agents based on current knowledge of pharmacogenetics, genomics, and physiological principles that are both universal and unique to the care of children at each stage in their development.

- Prescribes specific pharmacological agents and treatments based on clinical indicators, the child's status and needs, and results of diagnostic and laboratory tests.

- Provides the child (if age or developmentally appropriate) and family with information about diagnostic and laboratory results, as well as effects and potential adverse effects of proposed prescriptive therapies.

- Selects pharmacological and non-pharmacological treatments based on an evaluation of therapeutic and potential adverse effects.

- Provides information to the family regarding agents the child should refrain from taking because of potential adverse effects on the child.

- Provides the child (if age or developmentally appropriate) and family with information about costs, alternative treatments, and procedures as appropriate.

- Monitors current issues related to pharmacological agents, including off-label use and pediatric safe dosage for medications indicated for adults.

- Orders appropriate medications and treatments utilizing evidence-based guidelines and protocols.

Standard 6. Evaluation

The pediatric registered nurse evaluates progress toward attainment of outcomes.

Competencies

The pediatric registered nurse:

- Conducts a systematic, ongoing, and criterion-based evaluation of the outcomes in relation to structures and processes prescribed by the plan of care and indicated timeline.

- Collaborates with the child, family, healthcare providers, and others involved in the care or situation in the evaluation process.

- Evaluates, in partnership with the child and family, the effectiveness of planned strategies in relation to the child's responses and attainment of expected outcomes.

- Uses ongoing assessment data to revise the diagnoses, desired outcomes, plan, and implementation as needed.

- Disseminates results to the child, family, and others involved in accordance with federal and state regulations.

- Participates in assessing and assuring the responsible and appropriate use of interventions in order to minimize unwarranted or unwanted treatment and child suffering.

- Documents results of the evaluation.

- Refers to evaluation models to assist in evaluating outcomes.

Additional competencies for the advanced practice registered nurse

The advanced practice registered nurse:

- Evaluates diagnosis accuracy and the effectiveness of interventions and other variables in relation to the child's attainment of expected outcomes.

- Synthesizes results of the evaluation to determine the effect of the plan on children, providers, families, groups, communities, and institutions.

- Adapts the plan of care according to the evaluation of the child's response.

- Uses evaluation results to make or recommend process or structural changes, including policy, procedure, or protocol revision, as appropriate.

- Refers to best practice models to assist in evaluating outcomes.

- Synthesizes an evaluation, on a continual basis, as it relates to the effectiveness of care provided.

Standards of Professional Performance

Standard 7. Ethics
The pediatric registered nurse practices ethically.

Competencies
The pediatric registered nurse:

- Uses *Code of Ethics for Nurses with Interpretive Statements* (ANA 2015) to guide practice.

- Delivers care in a manner that preserves and protects the child's and family's autonomy, dignity, values, and rights.

- Delivers care in a nonjudgmental and nondiscriminatory manner that respects and values ethnic, racial, religious, and cultural diversity.

- Recognizes the centrality of the child and family as core members of the healthcare team.

- Maintains child and family confidentiality within legal and regulatory parameters.

- Enables children and families to participate in ethical decision-making processes.

- Maintains a therapeutic and professional relationship with appropriate role boundaries.

- Contributes to interprofessional teams or committees that address ethical questions, benefits, and outcomes.

- Reports abuse of patients' rights and incompetent, unethical, or illegal practice.

- Reports instances of illegal, unethical, or inappropriate behavior that endangers or jeopardizes the best interests of the child and family to administrators and the healthcare team.

Additional competencies for the advanced practice registered nurse

The advanced practice registered nurse:

- Ensures that the care provided is consistent with the child's and family's needs and values and is within codes of ethical practice.
- Informs the child (as appropriate) and family of the risks, benefits, and outcomes of healthcare regimens to support informed decision-making by the child and family.
- Makes decisions and initiates actions on behalf of children and their families in an ethical manner, taking into consideration the values of the child and family.
- Ensures informed consent or age-appropriate assent for procedures, treatment, and research, as appropriate.
- Serves as an advocate for the child and family in developing policies and providing care to the child and family.
- Contributes to the creation of individual and system responses to the resolution of ethical dilemmas.
- Advocates for a process of ongoing ethical inquiry into patient care practices where varying perspectives are acknowledged and validated.
- Participates in interprofessional teams that address ethical concerns, risks or considerations, benefits, and outcomes of patient care.
- Applies ethically sound solutions to complex issues related to individuals, populations, and systems of care.
- Identifies and communicates the risks, benefits, and outcomes of programs and decisions that may negatively affect healthcare delivery.

Standard 8. Education

The pediatric registered nurse attains knowledge and competence that reflect current nursing practice.

Competencies

The pediatric registered nurse:

- Participates in ongoing educational activities related to appropriate knowledge bases and professional issues.

- Demonstrates a commitment to lifelong learning through self-reflection and inquiry to address learning and personal growth needs.

- Seeks experiences that reflect evidence-based practice to maintain knowledge, skills, abilities, and judgment in clinical practice or role performance.

- Acquires knowledge and skills appropriate to the role, population, specialty, setting, or situation.

- Seeks formal and independent learning experiences to develop and maintain clinical and professional skills and knowledge.

- Identifies learning needs based on nursing knowledge, the various roles the nurse may assume, and the changing needs of the population.

- Participates in formal or informal consultations to address issues in nursing practice. Contributes to a work environment conducive to the education of healthcare professionals.

- Maintains professional records that provide evidence of competence and lifelong learning.

Additional competencies for the advanced practice registered nurse

The advanced practice registered nurse:

- Uses current evidence to expand clinical knowledge, skills, abilities, and judgment to enhance role performance and increase knowledge of professional issues.

- Participates in interprofessional educational experiences focusing on patient outcomes.

Standard 9. Evidence-based Practice and Research

The pediatric registered nurse integrates evidence and research findings into practice.

Competencies

The pediatric registered nurse:

- Utilizes the best available evidence, including research findings, to guide practice decisions.

- Contributes to the culture of safety by adhering to policy and procedures that demonstrate evidence-based best nursing practice.

- Protects the rights of all children and families involved in research studies with attention to:

  — Understanding that children are a vulnerable population and should receive special protection regarding confidentiality and exposure to risk.

  — Providing parents and guardians with additional support and education when providing consent for research that involves children.

  — Understanding the process of obtaining assent from children who are able to understand and provide agreement to participate (NAPNAP, 2010).

- Actively participates in research activities at various levels appropriate to the nurse's level of education, position, and practice environment. Such activities may include:

  — Identifying clinical problems or questions suitable for nursing research.

  — Identifying and recruiting potential candidates for enrollment.

  — Participating in data collection.

  — Participating in a formal committee or program.

  — Sharing research activities and findings with peers and others.

  — Conducting research.

  — Critically analyzing and interpreting evidence for application to practice.

- — Translating research findings and incorporating new knowledge in the development of policies, procedures, and standards of practice for the delivery of pediatric health care.

- — Incorporating research as a basis for learning.

Additional competencies for the advanced practice registered nurse

The advanced practice registered nurse:

- Contributes to nursing knowledge by conducting or synthesizing research that discovers, examines, and evaluates knowledge, theories, criteria, and creative approaches to improve healthcare practice and outcomes.

- Formally and informally disseminates research findings through practice, education, presentations, publications, consultation, and journal clubs.

- Promotes a climate of research and clinical inquiry.

Standard 10. Quality of Practice

The pediatric registered nurse contributes to quality nursing practice.

Competencies

The pediatric registered nurse:

- Demonstrates quality by documenting the application of the nursing process and evidence-based practice in a responsible, accountable, and ethical manner.

- Uses results of quality improvement activities to initiate changes in pediatric nursing practice and in the healthcare delivery system and disseminates results to others who may benefit.

- Uses creativity and innovation in pediatric nursing practice to improve care delivery to children and families.

- Incorporates new knowledge to initiate changes in nursing practice to support desired outcomes.

- Participates in quality improvement activities. Such activities may include:

  — Identifying nursing-sensitive indicators of pediatric nursing practice that are important for quality monitoring.

  — Using nursing-sensitive indicators developed to monitor quality and effectiveness of pediatric nursing practice.

  — Collecting data to monitor quality and effectiveness of pediatric nursing practice.

  — Analyzing quality data to identify opportunities for improving pediatric nursing practice.

  — Formulating recommendations to improve pediatric nursing practice and patient outcomes.

  — Developing, implementing, and evaluating activities, policies, procedures, and guidelines to improve the quality of pediatric nursing practice and patient care.

  — Participating on interprofessional teams to improve the care delivery process and patient outcomes.

  — Participating in efforts to maximize efficiencies and reduce financial burdens.

- — Analyzing factors related to patient safety, cost–benefit analysis, and service excellence, efficiency, and effectiveness.

- — Implementing processes to identify and address barriers within organizational systems.

- Provides leadership in the design and implementation of quality improvement initiatives.

- Designs innovations to effect change in practice environments and quality of nursing care rendered in relation to existing evidence.

- Obtains and maintains professional certification in advanced practice pediatric nursing.

- Participates in efforts to minimize financial burdens, reduce duplication of diagnostic services, and facilitate timely provision of services for children and their families.

- Identifies and removes barriers in organizational systems that may hinder the quality of pediatric nursing care.

Standard 11. Communication

The pediatric registered nurse communicates effectively in a variety of formats in all areas of practice.

Competencies

The pediatric registered nurse:

- Assesses communication format preferences of children, families, and colleagues.
- Assesses own communication skills in encounters with children, families, and colleagues.
- Identifies and communicates hazards and errors related to providing safe care to the pediatric patient.
- Maintains communication with other providers to minimize risks associated with transfers and transitions in care delivery.
- Contributes own professional perspective in discussions with the interprofessional team.
- Develops communication and conflict resolution skills.
- Maintains professional relationships with peers and colleagues.
- Contributes to a supportive and healthy work environment.
- Communicates effectively with the child, family, and colleagues.

Additional competencies for the advanced practice registered nurse

The advanced practice registered nurse:

- Leads the interprofessional team in developing effective communication patterns and conflict resolution.
- Promotes communication of information and advancement of the profession through writing, publishing, and preparing presentations for professional and lay audiences.
- Establishes effective communication modalities and formats between healthcare team members and the children and families for whom they care.

- Serves as a consultant for team members, families, and children who are having trouble communicating effectively.

- Advocates for health team members, families, and children, as appropriate, when conflicts in communication or decision-making arise.

Standard 12. Leadership
The pediatric registered nurse demonstrates leadership in the professional practice setting and the profession.

Competencies
The pediatric registered nurse:

- Provides oversight for nursing care given by others while retaining accountability for the quality of care given to the patient.
- Works to create and maintain healthy work environments in local, regional, national, or international communities.
- Abides by the vision, associated goals, and plan to implement and measure progress of an individual healthcare consumer or progress within the context of the healthcare organization.
- Demonstrates a commitment to professional development through continuous, lifelong learning.
- Demonstrates investment in others' success by teaching, mentoring, and precepting.
- Exhibits creativity and flexibility through times of change.
- Treats colleagues with respect, trust, and dignity.
- Mentors colleagues to advance nursing practice, the profession, and quality health care.
- Accepts accountability for errors by self and others, thereby creating a culture in which risk-taking is not only safe, but also expected.
- Inspires loyalty through valuing people as the most precious asset in an organization.
- Directs the coordination of care across settings and among care-givers, including overseeing licensed and unlicensed personnel in assigned or delegated tasks.
- Serves in key roles in the work setting by participating on committees, councils, and administrative teams.
- Promotes professional advancement through participation in professional organizations.
- Seeks ways to advance nursing autonomy and accountability.

- Participates in efforts to influence healthcare policy involving pediatric health care and the nursing profession.
- Shares knowledge and skills with peers, colleagues, and other stakeholders as evidenced by activities such as publications and presentations at meetings.

Additional competencies for the advanced practice registered nurse

The advanced practice registered nurse:

- Influences decision-making bodies to improve child health care, health services, and policies locally, regionally, nationally, and internationally.
- Provides direction to enhance the effectiveness of the interprofessional healthcare team.
- Promotes advanced practice nursing and role development by interpreting its role for patients, families, and the community.
- Mentors colleagues in the acquisition of clinical knowledge, skills, abilities, and judgment.
- Initiates and revises policies, protocols, and guidelines that reflect evidence-based practice and novel approaches in care management and address emerging trends.
- Designs innovations to effect change in practice and improve health outcomes.
- Contributes to an environment that is conducive to clinical education of other healthcare providers, including teaching, mentoring, and precepting.
- Contributes to others' professional development to improve child health care and to foster the profession's growth.

Standard 13. Collaboration

The pediatric registered nurse collaborates with the child, family, and others in the conduct of nursing practice.

Competencies

The pediatric registered nurse:

- Partners with others to effect change and positive outcomes through sharing knowledge.
- Promotes conflict management and engagement.
- Participates in building consensus or resolving conflict in the context of patient care.
- Applies group process and negotiation techniques.
- Adheres to standards and applicable codes of conduct that govern behavior among peers and colleagues to create a work environment that promotes cooperation, respect, and trust.
- Cooperates in creating a documented plan focused on outcomes and decisions related to care and delivery of services.
- Engages in teamwork and team-building processes.
- Documents referrals, including provision for continuity of care.
- Assists the family in identifying and accessing community resources, as appropriate, to support the family in the care of the child.
- Participates in interprofessional research teams and applies evidence to practice with children and families.

Additional competencies for the advanced practice registered nurse

The advanced practice registered nurse:

- Partners with other disciplines to enhance healthcare consumer outcomes through interprofessional activities, such as education, consultation, management, technological development, or research opportunities.
- Invites the contribution of the child, family, and team members in order to achieve optimal outcomes.

- Leads in establishing, improving, and sustaining collaborative relationships to achieve safe, quality health care for children and their families.

- Models expert practice to interprofessional team members and healthcare consumers.

- Actively participates in or provides guidance to research teams in discovery and application of evidence for nursing practice.

- Documents plan-of-care communications, rationales for plan-of-care changes, and collaborative discussions to improve child health outcomes.

- Participates on interprofessional teams that contribute to role development, advanced pediatric nursing practice, and health care.

Standard 14. Professional Practice Evaluation

The pediatric registered nurse evaluates her or his own nursing practice in relation to professional practice standards and guidelines and relevant statutes, rules, and regulations.

Competencies

The pediatric registered nurse:

- Evaluates own cultural and ethnic sensitivity when providing care.
- Engages in self-evaluation of practice on a regular basis, identifying areas of strength as well as areas in which professional development would be beneficial.
- Obtains informal feedback regarding own practice.
- Participates in systematic peer review as appropriate.
- Takes action to achieve goals identified during the evaluation process.
- Provides rationale for practice beliefs, decisions, and actions as part of the informal and formal evaluation processes.
- Applies knowledge of current professional practice standards, guidelines, statutes, rules, and regulations that affect the nursing care of children and families.
- Evaluates performance according to the standards of the nursing profession and the standards specific to pediatric nursing and associated regulatory bodies, taking action to improve practice.
- Analyzes the effectiveness of interventions, the incidence and types of complications, and child outcome data to improve practice.
- Takes action to achieve goals identified during performance appraisal and peer review, resulting in changes in practice and role performance.
- Synthesizes and uses the evaluation results to make recommended changes in guiding professional practice.

Additional competencies for the advanced practice registered nurse

The advanced practice registered nurse:

- Engages in a formal process seeking feedback regarding one's own practice from the child, family, peers, professional colleagues, and others.

- Actively participates in the process of monitoring the quality of one's own practice with periodic evaluation and plans to address deficiencies and continue improvement.

- Addresses patient safety with each client contact, incorporates safety standards in own practice, and periodically evaluates safety of the practice environment.

Standard 15. Resource Utilization

The pediatric registered nurse utilizes appropriate resources to plan and provide nursing services that are safe, effective, and financially responsible.

Competencies

The pediatric registered nurse:

- Evaluates factors such as patient safety, efficacy, efficiency, effectiveness, availability, cost, benefits, and impact on practice when deciding between practice options that would result in the same expected outcome.

- Assists the child and family in identifying and securing appropriate and available services to address their needs.

- Assigns or delegates tasks based on the needs and condition of the child, potential for benefit and/or harm, stability of the child's condition, complexity of the task, and predictability of the outcome.

- Assists the child and family in becoming informed consumers about treatment options and associated care, including the benefits, risks, and costs.

- Assists the family in identifying and accessing resources for pediatric patients requiring long-term, rehabilitative, palliative, and/or end-of-life care.

Additional competencies for the advanced practice registered nurse

The advanced practice registered nurse:

- Utilizes organizational and community resources to formulate interprofessional plans of care.

- Develops innovative solutions for child healthcare problems that address effective resource utilization and maintenance of quality.

- Develops evaluation strategies to demonstrate cost efficiency and effectiveness associated with pediatric nursing practice.

- Develops evaluation methods to measure patient safety and effectiveness for interventions and outcomes.

- Promotes activities that help others learn about benefits, risks, and costs of the plan of care.

- Initiates ongoing activities to analyze patient care systems in an effort to improve the quality of care provided to children and their families.

- Uses aggregate data, in collaboration with others, to develop or revise systems to avoid duplication of or gaps in service.

- Advocates for the elimination of barriers to care and supports the optimal level of care for the child and family.

- Develops innovative solutions and applies strategies to obtain appropriate resources for nursing initiatives.

- Secures organizational resources to ensure a work environment conducive to completing the identified plan of care and outcomes.

Standard 16. Environmental Health

The pediatric registered nurse practices in an environmentally safe and healthy manner.

Competencies

The pediatric registered nurse:

- Attains knowledge of environmental health concepts, such as implementation of environmental health strategies, with specific attention to the special needs of the health and well-being of children.

- Promotes a practice environment that reduces environmental health risks for coworkers, children, and families.

- Assesses the practice environment for factors such as sound, odor, noise, and light that threaten health.

- Advocates for the judicious and appropriate use of environmentally safe products in health care.

- Communicates environmental health risks and exposure reduction strategies to children and families, school systems, and communities.

- Utilizes scientific evidence to determine if a product or treatment is an environmental threat to children.

- Participates in strategies to promote healthy communities.

Additional competencies for the advanced practice registered nurse

The advanced practice registered nurse:

- Creates partnerships that promote sustainable environmental health policies and conditions.

- Analyzes the impact of social, political, and economic influences on the environment and pediatric health exposures.

- Critically evaluates the manner in which environmental health issues are presented by the popular media.

- Advocates for implementation of environmental principles for pediatric nursing practice.

- Supports nurses in advocating for and implementing environmental principles in pediatric nursing practice.

Standard 17. Advocacy

The pediatric registered nurse is an advocate for the pediatric patient and family.

Competencies

The pediatric registered nurse:

- Advocates for organizational, environmental, and practice changes to ensure that nursing care meets the unique health needs of children.

- Assists children and families to adjust to the changing healthcare environment.

- Protects the human and legal rights of the pediatric patient and family.

- Influences healthcare practice and policy in the care of children, families, and communities.

- Advocates that each child and family is provided with information in an appropriate language so they can make informed choices.

- Advocates for appropriate resources to assist the child and family in decision-making regarding healthcare choices.

- Advocates for the child, and works with families, social service agencies, and the courts when there is concern about child abuse, neglect, or other forms of family violence.

- Participates as a member of pediatric professional organizations.

- Advocates for local, state, and national policies to address the unique needs of children and families.

- Advocates for ethical policies and legislation that promote access to equitable and high-quality health care for children and families.

- Demonstrates an understanding of the laws that influence confidentiality in the provision of care (e.g., Health Insurance Portability Accountability Act [HIPAA] and Family Educational Rights and Privacy Act [FERPA]).

- Advocates for children and parents to assure they receive the rights guaranteed to them by federal law (e.g., Individuals with Disabilities Education Act [IDEA]).

Additional competencies for the advanced practice registered nurse

The advanced practice registered nurse:

- Advances the profession through enhancing public awareness and health professional familiarity with the advanced practice pediatric nursing role and scope of practice.

- Advocates for unrestricted access to quality, cost-effective care within healthcare agencies for children and families.

- Uses relevant policy specific to children to direct appropriate patient care and to eliminate financial and legislative restrictions that limit access to health care.

- Serves as an advocate for the unique needs of children and families within the healthcare system, including facilitating transitions across varying healthcare settings and the home.

References

All URLs were accessible as of September 10, 2015.

Advanced Practice Registered Nurses Consensus Work Group & National Council of State Boards of Nursing APRN Advisory Committee. (2008). *Consensus model for APRN regulation: Licensure, accreditation, certification, education.* Retrieved from https://www.ncsbn.org/ Consensus_Model_for_APRN_Regulation_July_2008.pdf

American Academy of Pediatrics, American Academy of Family Physicians, American College of Physicians, & Transitions Clinical Report Authoring Group. (2011). Supporting the health care transition from adolescence to adulthood in the medical home. *Pediatrics, 128*(1), 182–200. doi: 10.1542/peds.2011-0969

American Academy of Pediatrics, American Public Health Association, & National Resource Center for Health and Safety in Child Care and Early Education. (2011). *Caring for our children: National health and safety performance standards; Guidelines for early care and education programs (3rd ed.).* Elk Grove Village, IL: American Academy of Pediatrics; Washington, DC: American Public Health Association. Available from http://nrckids.org

American Academy of Pediatrics. (2012). Policy Statement: Palliative care for children. *Pediatrics.* 2000; *106*(2), 351–357. Reaffirmed February 2012.

American Academy of Pediatrics. (2013). Chronic conditions. Retrieved from http://www. healthychildren.org/english/health-issues/conditions/chronic/Pages/default.aspx

American Association of Colleges of Nursing. (2006). *The essentials of doctoral education for advanced nursing practice.* Washington, DC: Author.

American Association of Colleges of Nursing. (2008). *The essentials of baccalaureate education for professional nursing practice.* Washington, DC: Author. Retrieved from http://www.aacn.nche. edu/publications/order-form/baccalaureate-essentials

American Association of Colleges of Nursing. (2011). *The essentials of master's education for advanced practice nursing.* Washington, DC: Author. Retrieved from http://www.aacn.nche. edu/publications/order-form/masters-essentials

American Association of Nurse Practitioners. (May 2015). [Map of U.S. nurse practitioner environments]. *2015 Nurse practitioner state practice environment.* Retrieved from http:// www.aanp.org/images/documents/state-leg-reg/stateregulatorymap.pdf

American Nurses Association. (2001). *Code of ethics for nurses with interpretive statements.* Silver Spring, MD: Author.

American Nurses Association. (2004). *Nursing: Scope and standards of practice.* Silver Spring, MD: Author.

American Nurses Association. (2010a). ANA position statement: The nurse's role in ethics and human rights: Protecting and promoting individual worth, dignity, and human rights in practice settings. Retrieved from http://www.nursingworld.org/MainMenuCategories/EthicsStandards/Ethics-Position-Statements/-Nurses-Role-in-Ethics-and-Human-Rights.pdf

American Nurses Association. (2010b). *Nursing: Scope and standards of practice* (2nd ed.). Silver Spring, MD: Author.

American Nurses Association. (2010c). *Nursing's social policy statement: The essence of the profession* (3rd ed.). Silver Spring, MD: Author.

American Nurses Association & Society of Pediatric Nurses. (2003). *Scope and standards of pediatric nursing practice*. Silver Spring, MD: Nursesbooks.org.

American Public Health Association, Inc. (1955). *Health supervision of young children*. New York, NY: Author.

Association of Camp Nurses. (2005). *The scope and standards of camp nursing practice* (2nd ed.). Bernidji, MN: Author.

Blum, R. W., Garel, D., Hodgeman, C. H., Jorissen, T. W., Okinow, N. A., Orr, D. P., & Slap, G. B. (1993).Transition from child-centered to adult health-care systems for adolescents with chronic conditions: A position paper of the Society for Adolescent Medicine. *The Journal of Adolescent Health, 14*(7), 570–576.

Brewer, K. C. (2011). Quality recognition and the healthcare home. *Nursing Management, 42*(4), 10–14.

Butts, J. B., & Rich, K.L. (2013). *Nursing ethics: Across the curriculum and into practice* (3rd ed.). Boston, MA: Jones and Bartlett.

Caplan, G. (1961). *An approach to community mental health*. New York, NY: Grune and Stratton.

Center for Healthcare Transition Improvement. (2012). [Chart comparison of six core elements of transition]. *Six core elements of health care transition 2.0.* Retrieved from http://www.gottransition.org/resourceGet.cfm?id=206

Centers for Disease Control and Prevention. (2011a). 2011 National immunization survey. Retrieved from http://www.cdc.gov/nchs/nis/data_files.htm

Centers for Disease Control and Prevention. (2011b). Injury center: Violence prevention: Youth violence national and state statistics at a glance. Retrieved from http://www.cdc.gov/ViolencePrevention/pdf/YV-DataSheet-a.pdf

Centers for Disease Control and Prevention. (2012a). *Health, United States, 2012: With special feature on emergency care*. Retrieved from http://www.cdc.gov/nchs/data/hus/hus12.pdf

Centers for Disease Control and Prevention. (2012b). National, state, and local area vaccination coverage among children aged 19-35 Months – United States, 2011. *Morbidity and Mortality Weekly Report, 61*(35). Retrieved from http://www.cdc.gov/mmwr/pdf/wk/mm6135.pdf

Centers for Disease Control and Prevention. (2012c). Vital signs: Unintentional injury deaths among persons aged 0-19 Years – United States, 2000-2009. *Morbidity and Mortality Weekly Report, 61*(15). Retrieved from http://www.cdc.gov/mmwr/preview/mmwrhtml/mm61e0416a1.htm

Chaplic, K. C., & Allen, P. J. (2013). Best practices to identify gay, lesbian, bisexual or questioning youth in primary care. *Pediatric Nursing, 39*(2), 99–103.

Children's Defense Fund. (2010). *State of America's children*. Retrieved from http://www.childrensdefense.org/child-research-data-publications/data/the-state-of-america s-children-2010-report-health.pdf

Children's Hospital Association. (2013). All children need children's hospitals [pamphlet]. Retrieved from http://www.upstate.edu/gch/pdf/allchildren.pdf

Consensus Panel on Genetic/Genomic Nursing Competencies. (2008). *Essential nursing competencies and curricula guidelines for genetics and genomics* (2nd ed.). Silver Spring, MD: American Nurses Association.

Cowell, J., & Swartwout, K. (2006). Healthcare home: Ensuring access to a regular healthcare provider. In M. Craft-Rosenberg & M. Krajicek (Eds.), *Nursing excellence for children and families* (pp. 23–40). New York, NY: Springer Publishing Co.

Craft-Rosenberg, M., & Krajicek, M. (Eds.). (2006). *Nursing excellence for children and families.* New York, NY: Springer Publishing Co.

Crowley, R., Wolfe, I., Lock, K., & McKee, M. (2011). Improving the transition between pediatric and adult healthcare: A systematic review. *Archives of Disease in Childhood, 96*, 548–553.

Davis, A. M., Brown, R. F., Taylor, J. L., Epstein, R. A., & McPheeters, M. L. (2014). Transition care for children with special health care needs. *Pediatrics, 134*(5), 900–908.

Dellon, E. S., Jones, P. D., Martin, N. B., Kelly, M., Kim, S., Freeman, K., … Shaheen, N. J. (2013). Health care transition from pediatric to adult-focused gastroenterology in patients with eosinophilic esophagitis. *Diseases of the Esophagus, 26*(1), 7–13.

Eaton, D. K., Kann, L., Kinchen, S., Shanklin, S., Flint, K. H., Hawkins, J., … Wechsler, H. (2012). Youth risk behavior surveillance — United States, 2011. *Morbidity and Mortality Weekly Report. Surveillance Summary, 61*(4), 1–162.

Fernandes, S. M., O'Sullivan-Oliveira, J., Landzberg, M. J., Khairy, P., Melvin, P., Sawicki, G. S., … Fishman, L. N. (2014). Transition and transfer of adolescents and young adults with pediatric onset chronic disease: the patient and parent perspective. *Journal of Pediatric Rehabilitation Medicine, 7*(1), 43–51.

Fieldston, E. S., & Altschuler, S. M. (2013). Implications of the growing use of freestanding children's hospitals. *JAMA Pediatrics, 167*(2), 190–192.

Finocchio, L. J., Dower, C. M., McMahon, T., Gragnola, C. M., & Taskforce on Health Care Workforce Regulation. (1995). *Reforming health care workforce regulation: Policy considerations for the 21st century.* San Francisco, CA: Pew Health Professions Commission.

Fowler, M. (2010). *Guide to the code of ethics for nurses: Interpretation and application.* Silver Spring, MD: Nursebooks.org.

Guilday, P. (2000). School nursing practice today: Implications for the future. *Journal of School Nursing, 16*(5), 25–31. doi: 10.1177/105984050001600504

Hait, E., Arnold, J. H., & Fishman, L. N. (2006). Educate, communicate, anticipate-practical recommendations for transitioning adolescents with IBD to adult health care. *Inflammatory Bowel Diseases, 12*(1), 70–73. doi: 10.1097/01.MIB.0000194182.85047.6a

Hanna, H., Matthews, R., Cross, G. W., Kotch, J. Blanchard, T., & Cosby, A. G. (2012). Use of paid child health care consultants in early care and education settings: Results of a national study comparing provision of health care screening services among Head Start and non-Head Start Centers. *Journal of Pediatric Health Care, 26*(6), 427–435. doi: 10.1016/j.pedhc.2011.05.008

Hartigan, C. (2011). APRN Regulation: The licensure-certification interface. *AACN Advanced Critical Care, 22*(1), 50–65.

Health Resources and Services Administration. (2013). School-based health centers. Retrieved from: http://www.hrsa.gov/ourstories/schoolhealthcenters/

Henderson, V. (1964). The nature of nursing. *American Journal of Nursing, 64*(8), 62–68.

Institute for Patient- and Family-Centered Care. (2010). Frequently asked questions. Retrieved from http://www.ipfcc.org/faq.html

Institute of Medicine. (2001). *Crossing the quality chasm: A new health system for the 21st century.* Washington, DC: National Academies Press.

Institute of Medicine. (2011). *Future of nursing: Leading change, advancing health.* Washington, DC: National Academies Press.

Kim, Y. Y., Gauvreau, K., Bacha, E. A., Landzberg, M. J., & Benavidez, O. J. (2011). Risk factors for death after adult congenital heart surgery in pediatric hospitals. *Circulation. Cardiovascular Quality and Outcomes, 4,* 433–439.

Kovacs, A. H., & Verstappen, A. (2011). The whole adult congenital heart disease patient. *Progress in Cardiovascular Diseases, 53,* 247–253.

Kuo, D. Z., Houtrow, H., Arango, P., Kuhlthau, K. A., Simmons, J. M., & Neff, J.M. (2012). Family centered care: Current applications and future directions in pediatric health care. *Maternal and Child Health Journal, 16*(2), 297–305.

Lemly, D. C., Weitzman, E. R., & O'Hare, K. (2013). Advancing healthcare transitions in the medical home: Tools for providers, families and adolescents with special healthcare needs. *Current Opinion in Pediatrics, 25*(4), 439–446.

Leung, Y., Heyman, M. B., & Mahadevan, U. (2011). Transitioning the adolescent inflammatory bowel disease patient: Guidelines for the adult and pediatric gastroenterologist. *Inflammatory Bowel Disease, 17*(10), 2169–2173.

Lofquist, D., Lugaila, T., O'Connell, M., & Feliz, S. (2012*). Households and families: 2010.* Washington, DC: U.S. Census Bureau. Retrieved from http://www.census.gov/prod/cen2010/briefs/c2010br-14.pdf

Looman, W. S., O'Conner-Von, S., & Lindeke, L. (2008). Caring for children with special health care needs and their families: What advanced practice nurses need to know. *The Journal for Nurse Practitioners, 4*(7), 512–517.

Mastro, K. A., Flynn, L., & Preuster, C. (2014). Patient and family centered care: A call to action for new knowledge and innovation. *Journal of Nursing Administration, 44*(9), 446–451.

Melnyk, B., & Fineout-Overholt, E. (Eds.). (2010). *Evidence-based practice in nursing and health care* (2nd ed.). Philadelphia, PA: Lippincott, Williams and Wilkins.

National Association of Clinical Nurse Specialists. (2004). *Statement on clinical nurse specialist practice and education* (2nd ed.). Harrisburg, PA: Author.

National Association of Neonatal Nurses. (2006). *Education standards for neonatal nurse practitioner programs.* Glenview, IL: Author.

National Association of Neonatal Nurses. (2013). *Neonatal nursing scope and standards of practice* (2nd ed.). Silver Spring, MD: American Nurses Association.

National Association of Pediatric Nurse Practitioners. (2004). *Scope and standards of practice: Pediatric nurse practitioner (PNP).* New York, NY: Author.

National Association of Pediatric Nurse Practitioners. (2008a). NAPNAP position statement on age parameters for PNP practice. *Journal of Pediatric Health Care, 22*(3), e1–e2. doi: 10.1016.j.pedhc.2008.02.007

National Association of Pediatric Nurse Practitioners. (2008b). *NAPNAP research agenda 2008-2013: Priorities for evidence in practice.* New York, NY: Author.

National Association of Pediatric Nurse Practitioners. (2009). NAPNAP position statement on pediatric health care/medical home: Key issues on delivery, reimbursement, and leadership. *Journal of Pediatric Health Care, 25*(3), 23A–24A. doi: 10.1016/j.pedhc.2009.02.005

National Association of Pediatric Nurse Practitioners. (2010a). NAPNAP position statement on the acute care nurse practitioner. *Journal of Pediatric Health Care, 25*(3), e11–e12. doi: 10.1016/j.pedhc.2010.12.004

National Association of Pediatric Nurse Practitioners. (2010b). NAPNAP position statement on protection of children involved in research studies. *Journal of Pediatric Health Care, 2*(1), 17A–18A. doi: 10.1016/j.pedhc.2009.08.012

National Association of Pediatric Nurse Practitioners. (2011). Health risks and needs of lesbian, gay, bisexual, transgender, and questioning adolescents position statement. *Journal of Pediatric Health Care, 25*(6), A9–A10. doi: 10.1016/j.pedhc.2011.07.002

National Association of Pediatric Nurse Practitioners. (2012). NAPNAP position statement on access to care. *Journal of Pediatric Health Care, 26*(2), 21A–23A. doi: 10.1016/j.pedhc.2011.11.003

National Association of Pediatric Nurse Practitioners. (2013). NAPNAP position statement on school-based health care. *Journal of Pediatric Health Care, 27*(3), A15–A16. doi: 10.1016/j.pedhc.2013.01.004

National Association of School Nurses. (2012a). *Chronic health conditions managed by school nurses.* Retrieved from http://www.nasn.org/PolicyAdvocacy/PositionPapersandReports/NASNPositionStatementsFullView/tabid/462/ArticleId/17/Chronic-Health-Conditions-Managed-by-School-Nurses-Revised-January-2012

National Association of School Nurses. (2012b). *Education, licensure, and certification of school nurses.* Retrieved from http://www.nasn.org/PolicyAdvocacy/PositionPapersandReports/NASNPositionStatementsFullView/tabid/462/smid/824/ArticleID/26/Default.aspx

National Association of School Nurses & American Nurses Association. (2005). *School nursing scope and standards of practice.* Silver Spring, MD: American Nurses Association.

National Center for Complementary and Alternative Medicine. (2013). *Complementary, alternative, or integrative health: What's in a name?* Retrieved from http://nccam.nih.gov/health/whatiscam?nav=gsa

National Council of State Boards of Nursing. (2012). *Changes in healthcare professions' scope of practice: Legislative considerations.* Retrieved from https://www.ncsbn.org/4625.htm

National Hospice and Palliative Care Organization. (2012). *Concurrent care.* Retrieved from http://www.nhpco.org/sites/default/files/public/ChiPPS/Continuum_Briefing.pdf

National Organization of Nurse Practitioner Faculties. (2013). *Population-focused nurse practitioner competencies: Family/across the lifespan, neonatal, acute care pediatric, primary care pediatric, psychiatric-mental health, & women's health/gender-related.* Washington, DC: Author.

National Panel for Acute Care Nurse Practitioner Competencies. (2004). *Acute care nurse practitioner competencies.* Washington, DC: Author.

Nehring, W. M., Roth, S. P., Natvig, D., Betz, C. L., Savage, T., & Krajicek, M. (2004). *Intellectual and developmental disabilities nursing: Scope and standards of practice.* Silver Springs, MD: American Nurses Association.

Noonan, J. A. (2004). A history of pediatric specialties: The development of pediatric cardiology. *Pediatric Research, 56*(2), 298–306.

Oberg, C. N. (2012). Embracing international children's rights: From principles to practice. *Clinical Pediatrics, 51*(7), 619–624. doi: 10.1177/0009922811417302

O'Sullivan-Oliveira, J., Fernandes, S., Borges, L., & Fishman, L. (2014). Transition of pediatric patients to adult care, an analysis of provider perceptions across discipline and role. *Pediatric Nursing, 40*(3), 113–120.

Pelletier, L. R., & Stichler, J. F. (2014). Ensuring patient and family engagement, a professional nurse's toolkit. *Journal of Nursing Care Quality, 15*(2), 110–114.

Philpott, J. R. (2011). Transitional care in inflammatory bowel disease. *Gastroenterology & Hepatology, 7*(1), 26–32.

Pridham, K. F. (1993). Anticipatory guidance of parents of new infants: Potential contribution of the internal working model construct. *Image: Journal of Nursing Scholarship, 25*(1), 49–56.

Putman, G. (2014). Nurses, advocacy and the impact of healthcare reform on children. *Journal of Pediatric Nursing, 29*(2), 189–190.

Rosenblum, R. K., & Sprague-McRae, J. (2013). Using principles of quality and safety education for nurses in school nurse continuing education. *Journal of School Nursing* (Epub ahead of print). doi: 10.1177/1059840513489710

Sackett, D. L., Straus, S. E., Richardson, W. S., Rosenberg, W., & Haynes, R. B. (2000). *Evidence-based medicine: How to practice and teach EBM.* Edinburgh, UK: Churchill Livingstone.

Safriet, B. J. (2011). Federal options for maximizing the value of advanced practice nurses in providing quality, cost-effective health care: Appendix H. In Institute of Medicine (Ed.), *The future of nursing: Leading change, advancing health* (pp. 443–475). Washington, DC: National Academies Press. Retrieved from http://www.nap.edu/catalog/12956.html

Silver, H. K., Ford, L. C., & Stearly, S. G. (1967). A program to increase health care for children: The pediatric nurse practitioner. *Pediatrics, 39*(5),756–760.

Society of Pediatric Nurses. (2004). *The role of the staff nurse in protecting children and families involved in research.* http://www.pedsnurses.org/pdfs/downloads/gid,68/index.pdf [no longer available online]

Society of Pediatric Nurses. (2014). *Position statement on child health content in the undergraduate curriculum.* Retrieved from http://www.pedsnurses.org/p/cm/ld/fid=57&tid=28&sid=67

Society of Pediatric Nurses, National Association of Pediatric Nurse Practitioners, & American Nurses Association. (2008). *Pediatric nursing: Scope and standards of practice.* Silver Spring, MD: American Nurses Association.

Taylor, M. K. (2006). Mapping the literature of pediatric nursing. *Journal of the Medical Library Association, 94*(2), E128–136.

U.S. Department of Health and Human Services. (2011). *HHS action plan to reduce racial and ethnic health disparities: A nation free of disparities in health and health care.* Washington, DC: Author.

U.S. Department of Health and Human Services. Health Services and Resources Administration. (2013). The Affordable Care Act and Health Centers. (HRSA fact sheet). Retrieved from http://www.hrsa.gov/about/news/2012tables/healthcentersacafactsheet.pdf

U.S. Department of Health and Human Services, Child Welfare Information Gateway. (n.d.). Philosophy and key elements of family-centered practice. Retrieved from https://www.childwelfare.gov/famcentered/philosophy.cfm

U.S. Department of Health and Human Services, Health Resources and Services Administration & Maternal and Child Health Bureau. (2004). *The national survey of children with special health care needs chartbook 2001.* Rockville, MD: U.S. Department of Health and Human Services.

U.S. Department of Health and Human Services. (2015). About the law. Retrieved from http://www.hhs.gov/healthcare/rights/

U.S. Department of Health and Human Services, Health Resources and Services Administration, & Maternal and Child Health Bureau. (2008). *The national survey of children with special health care needs chartbook 2005-2006.* Rockville, MD: U.S. Department of Health and Human Services.

Ventola, C. L. (2010). Current issues regarding complementary and alternative medicine (CAM) in the U.S., Part 1: The widespread use of CAM and the need for better-informed health care professionals to provide patient counseling. *Pharmacy and Therapeutics, 35*(8), 461–468.

Woodring, B. C., & Pridham, K. F. (Eds.). (1998). *Standards and guidelines for pre-licensure and early professional education for the nursing care of children and their families* (Revised). Document #H112R77. Washington, DC: DHHS/PHS.

World Health Organization. (2007). *International classification of functioning, disability and health—Children and youth version (ICF–CY).* Geneva: WHO.

Appendix A
Comprehensive List of Assessment Criteria for Pediatric Nursing

This list is to be used in conjunction with the final competency for Standard 1, Assessment, on page 46.

- *Physical assessment* may include but not be limited to:
  - Height, length, weight (current and pre-illness), and body mass index (BMI).
  - Vital signs including pain assessment.
  - Age-appropriate physical screening including, but not limited to, vision, hearing, and scoliosis screening.
  - Tanner staging of pubertal development.
  - Nutritional status.
  - Physical examination.
  - Age-appropriate measurements such as head, chest, and waist circumference.
- *Behavioral assessment* may include but not be limited to:
  - Tolerance of the physical examination or procedures.
  - Affect and activity.
  - Interactions with adults and peers.
  - Behavioral differences across settings (home, school, clinic, hospital).
- *Developmental assessment* may include but not be limited to:
  - Personal characteristics and social skills.
  - Language.
  - Fine motor and adaptive.

- — Gross motor.

- — Cognitive.

- — Emotional and mental health.

- — Temperament.

- — Moral development.

- — Performance at school and learning style.

- *Family assessment* may include:

  - — Determining whom the child lives with.

  - — Familial strengths and areas for improvement.

  - — Cultural background.

  - — Ethnic background.

  - — Socioeconomic background.

  - — Mental health issues.

  - — Religious or spiritual background.

  - — Coping strategies.

  - — Learning style preferences, including language, of family for receiving information and support.

  - — Injury prevention and safety practices.

  - — Interactions with child's teachers or other adults outside of the home.

  - — Ways the family can collaborate in providing the child's health care.

- *Health history* may include but not be limited to:

  - — Birth history (age-appropriate).

  - — Growth and developmental milestones.

  - — Past medical illnesses, hospitalizations, or surgeries.

  - — Medications and allergies.

  - — Family history, including three-generation genogram and known congenital abnormalities or associated conditions.

  - — Mental or emotional disabilities, metabolic problems, and chronic health problems.

- Accidents or injuries.
- Educational needs related to maximizing the child's health.
- Behavioral patterns and individual strengths.
- Communicable or childhood diseases.
- Exposure to hazardous agents.
- Dietary habits and typical intake history.
- Growth parameters as compared with normal for age.
- Significant trends in weight gain or loss.
- Immunization status.
- Sexual history (age-appropriate).
- Substance abuse history (age-appropriate).
- Engagement in high-risk activities (smoking, drugs or alcohol, body piercing or tattoos, sexual activity, or performance-enhancing drugs).
- Experience with pain and pain management techniques.
- School history (age-appropriate).
- Elimination patterns.
- Sleep habits and sleep patterns.
- Information that family member sees as significant.
- Family or other adult observations of the child.
- Strengths of the child and family.
- Any significant stressors, comforting and coping strategies.
- Relationships with the family, including potential for abuse.
- Socioeconomic, cultural, spiritual, and environmental factors.
- Peer relationships.
- Travel history.

Appendix B
Pediatric Nursing: Scope and Standards of Practice (2008)

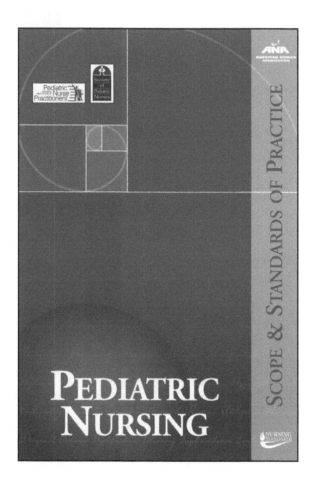

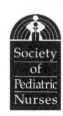

PEDIATRIC NURSING:

SCOPE AND STANDARDS

OF PRACTICE

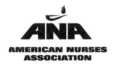

AMERICAN NURSES ASSOCIATION
SILVER SPRING, MARYLAND
2008

ACKNOWLEDGMENTS

The unified *Pediatric Nursing: Scope and Standards of Practice* was developed by a work group composed of members from both the National Association of Pediatric Nurse Practitioners and the Society of Pediatric Nurses, in collaboration with the American Nurses Association. It addresses pediatric nursing practice at all levels and in all settings and can be used by clinicians, educators, public, regulators, and legislators.

Joint Scope and Standards Writing Work Group Members

Lynn Mohr, MS, PCNS-BC, CPN *(co-Chair, SPN)*
Advocate Hope Children's Hospital, Oak Lawn, IL
Martha K. Swartz, PhD, RN, CPNP *(co-Chair, NAPNAP)*
Yale University School of Nursing, New Haven, CT
Patricia Clinton, PhD, RN, CPNP, FAANP *(NAPNAP; Ex-Officio)*
University of Iowa College of Nursing, Iowa City, IA
Linda Kollar, MSN, CPNP *(NAPNAP)*
Cincinnati Children's Hospital Medical Center, Cincinnati, OH
Carolyn Jaramillo de Montoya, MSN, CPNP *(NAPNAP ; Ex-Officio)*
University of New Mexico, College of Nursing, Albuquerque, NM
Sandy Mott, PhD, RN, BC *(SPN; Ex-Officio)*
Boston College, William F. Connell School of Nursing, Chestnut Hill, MA
LaDonna Northington, DNS, RN, BC, CCRN *(SPN)*
University of Mississippi, School of Nursing, Jackson, MS
Elizabeth Preze, MSN, CPNP PC/AC *(NAPNAP)*
Children's Memorial Hospital, Chicago, IL
Jo Ann Serota, MSN, RN, CPNP *(NAPNAP; Ex-Officio)*
Ambler Pediatrics, Ambler, PA
Linda Youngstrom, DNSc, RN *(SPN)*
Children's Hospital of Philadelphia, Philadelphia, PA
Joal Hill, JD, MPH, PhD *(Ethics consultant)*
Director of Research Ethics Advocate Healthcare, Park Ridge, IL

Joint Scope and Standards Review Panel Work Group Members

Ruth Bindler, PhD, RNC *(SPN)*
Washington State University, Spokane, WA
Mary Bjorklund, MSN, RN, CPN *(SPN)*
Lonestar College, Kingwood, TX

iii

Appendix B. Pediatric Nursing: Scope and Standards of Practice (2008)

Kristen Bonner, RN *(SPN)*
Saint Vincent Healthcare, Billings, MT
Nan Gaylord, PhD, RN, CPNP *(NAPNAP)*
University of Tennessee, Knoxville, TN
Eva Gomez, MSN, RN *(SPN)*
Children's Hospital Boston, Boston, MA
Catherine Goodhue, MSN, RN, CPNP *(NAPNAP)*
Childrens Hospital Los Angeles, Los Angeles, CA
Peg Harrison, MS, RN, CPNP *(SPN)*
Pediatric Nursing Certification Board, Gaithersburg, MD
Jean Ivey, DSN, CPNP *(NAPNAP)*
University of Alabama at Birmingham, School of Nursing,
Birmingham, AL
Patricia Jackson Allen, MS, RN, PNP, FAAN *(NAPNAP)*
Yale University School of Nursing, New Haven, CT
Andrea M. Kline, RN, MS, CPNP-AC/PC, FCCM *(NAPNAP)*
Children's Memorial Hospital, Chicago, IL
Anne Longo, MBA, BSN, RN-BC *(SPN)*
Cincinnati Children's Hospital, Cincinnati, OH
Debby Mason, MSN, CNP *(SPN)*
Cincinnati Children's Hospital, Cincinnati, OH
Cherie McCann, MSN, RN, BC, CPN *(SPN)*
Pacific Lutheran University, School of Nursing, Tacoma, WA
Armstrong Atlantic State University, Department of Nursing,
Savannah, GA
Sherry McCoy, MSN, RN, CPNP *(NAPNAP)*
Kaiser Permanente, Garden Grove, CA
Barbara Meeks, MSN, MBA, RN *(SPN)*
MCGHealth Children's Medical Center, Augusta, GA
Melissa Reider-Demer, MSN, CPNP *(NAPNAP)*
Childrens Hospital Los Angeles, Los Angeles, CA
Lizabeth Sumner, RN, BSN, RN *(SPN)*
The Elizabeth Hospice, Escondido, CA
Phyllis Thatcher, RN *(SPN)*
Brenner Children's Hospital, Winston-Salem, NC

Joint Scope and Standards Participating Organizations

American Nurses Association (ANA)
National Association of Pediatric Nurse Practitioners (NAPNAP)
Society of Pediatric Nurses (SPN)

iv

American Nurses Association Staff

Carol J. Bickford, PhD, RN-BC – Content editor
Yvonne Humes, MLB – Project coordinator
Maureen Cones – Legal counsel

NAPNAP and SPN Staff

Dolores C. Jones, EdD, RN, CPNP, CAE *(NAPNAP)*
Karen KellyThomas, PhD, RN, FAAN, CAE *(NAPNAP)*
Belinda Puetz, PhD, RN *(SPN)*

About NAPAP

The National Association of Pediatric Nurse Practitioners (NAPNAP) is the professional association for pediatric nurse practitioners and other advanced practice nurses who provide health care for children and families. NAPNAP promotes optimal health for children through leadership, practice, advocacy, education and research. (http://www.napnap.org/)

About SPN

The Society of Pediatric Nurses (SPN) is the premiere pediatric nursing association providing international leadership and promoting the specialty of pediatric nursing in practice, education, and research. The society influences public policy and legislation through collaboration with other nursing organizations and professional organizations dedicated to promoting and improving the health of children. (https://www.pedsnurses.org/)

Descriptions and websites of these groups are in Appendix A, which begins on pg. 85.

Appendix B. Pediatric Nursing: Scope and Standards of Practice (2008)

v

CONTENTS

Appendix B. Pediatric Nursing: Scope and Standards of Practice (2008)

The content in this appendix is not current and is of historical significance only.

ix

PREFACE

Pediatric nursing is the protection, promotion, and optimization of health and abilities for children of newborn age through young adulthood. Utilizing a family-centered care approach, pediatric nursing includes the prevention of illness and injury, the alleviation of suffering through the diagnosis and treatment of the child's response, and advocacy in the care of children and families.

The primary purpose of a scope of practice statement is to protect the public and enhance consumers' access to competent healthcare services. It is also incumbent upon a profession to define the scope and standards of practice within that profession, and to ensure that scope of practice changes reflect the evolution of abilities within the particular healthcare discipline. This publication is the result of a unique, two-year collaborative effort in which members of the National Association of Pediatric Nurse Practitioners (NAPNAP) joined with representatives of the Society of Pediatric Nurses (SPN) and the American Nurses Association (ANA) to launch a new, unified scope and standards of pediatric nursing practice document for the benefit of children, the public, and all the nurses who care for them.

Prior to our efforts, there were two pediatric nursing scope and standards documents available to practitioners, the nursing profession, legislators, regulators, accrediting bodies, and the public. This new publication is based on the ground-breaking work that was put forth in the original *Scope and Standards of Pediatric Nursing Practice* (ANA & SPN, 2003), the *Scope and Standards of Practice: Pediatric Nurse Practitioner (PNP)* (NAPNAP, 2004b) as well as *Nursing: Scope and Standards of Practice* (ANA, 2004). By developing a unified document, NAPNAP and SPN seek to reduce confusion and create a new and improved set of standards that addresses all areas of pediatric nursing practice.

The history of the pediatric specialty within nursing can be traced back to the very early part of the twentieth century. Articles addressing the needs of children appeared in nursing journals as far back as 1906, and the first pediatric nursing text was published in 1923 (Connolly, 2005). General pediatric nursing continued to grow as a specialty throughout the 1900s, and the latter part of the century witnessed the development of professional pediatric nursing organizations, the

xi

availability of certification, and the development of standards (Taylor, 2006).

In 1964, Drs. Loretta C. Ford (a pediatric nurse) and Henry K. Silver (a pediatrician) worked together to launch the first PNP program. In that same year, a PNP program was also begun at Massachusetts General Hospital in Boston. The programs' goals were to expand the role of the pediatric nurse to fill gaps in health care for children. The concept was quickly adopted by others, and by 1980 over 300 PNP programs existed (Murphy, 1990). In 1973, the National Association of Pediatric Nurse Associates and Practitioners was formed. (The word "associates" was later dropped from the official NAPNAP name.) Since its inception, NAPNAP has been a leader in many areas for PNPs including education, research, professional development, advocacy, and practice.

SPN was founded in the mid-1980s as a more broad-based pediatric nursing organization whose members now include staff nurses, school and outpatient nurses, clinical nurse specialists, practitioners, administrators, educators, and researchers (Miles, 1996). The Society offers its members the opportunity to interact with colleagues of similar interests and to share ideas, research, and expertise. Through collaborative efforts with other nursing, medical, child health, and child health advocacy groups, the Society also influences legislation, health policy, and public education.

With the evident commonalities in the missions, goals, and activities of both NAPNAP and SPN, it became clear that for both organizations to collaborate and undertake the development of a comprehensive scope and standards document for pediatric nursing would be of benefit to pediatric nurses in all areas of practice, and also provide a unified voice to the public.

In our writing, we were also guided by several assumptions recently described in the monograph *Changes in Healthcare Professions' Scope of Practice: Legislative Consideration* (Association of Social Work Boards et al., 2007). This work, put forth by an interdisciplinary panel of health professional groups (including nursing, social work, medicine, pharmacy, and physical and occupational therapy) suggests the following:

(1) public protection should have top priority in scope of practice decisions;

(2) changes in scope of practice are inherent in our current healthcare system;

xii

(3) collaboration among healthcare providers should be the professional norm; and

(4) overlap among professions is necessary.

That is: no one profession owns a skill or activity in and of itself. Rather, it is the entire scope of activities within a practice that makes a particular profession unique.

Pediatric Nursing: Scope and Standards of Practice describes the scope of activities inherent in pediatric nursing. It describes aspects of competent nursing care and professional performance which are measurable, can be evaluated, and are common to nurses engaged in the care of children and their families based on their generalist or advanced practice role. This one document speaks to the standards of professional performance in all areas of pediatric nursing practice and will serve as a resource not only for nursing faculty and students but also for healthcare providers, researchers, and those involved in funding, legal, policy, and regulatory activities.

We are optimistic that you will find *Pediatric Nursing: Scope and Standards of Practice* useful to you, not only in your daily practice but also when answering larger questions relating to education, public policy and advocacy. We also hope this document will reinforce the inclusion of pediatric nursing as an important component in the plans of study for generalist nurses. The health of our nation's children is dependent on well-educated, qualified, and competent nurses who have the requisite knowledge and skill to care for our more than 71 million children and adolescents living in the United States today.

It took a large team to develop this unified voice. In particular, we would like to acknowledge other members of the writing work group: Linda Kollar and Elizabeth Preze of NAPNAP, and LaDonna Northington, Linda Youngstrom, Sandy Mott, and Belinda Puetz of SPN. Thanks also to Carolyn Jaramillo de Montoya, Patricia Clinton, Jo Ann Serota, Karen KellyThomas, Dolores Jones, and Jennifer Knorr at NAPNAP. After our initial writing, a draft was sent to a Review Panel Work Group consisting of members of both NAPNAP and SPN. Following this, a draft was posted on the ANA, NAPNAP, and SPN web sites for public comment. To all who participated in these important steps, thank you!

In many ways, the work of writing pediatric nursing's scope and standards of practice is an ongoing process, as our profession continues to

xiii

Appendix B. Pediatric Nursing: Scope and Standards of Practice (2008)

evolve and the healthcare climate changes. Your input will be invaluable, and we encourage you to be an active part of this process when, in a few short years, we will have another opportunity to update our scope and standards of practice.

Lynn Mohr, MS, RN PCNS-BC CPN (Co-chair, SPN
Martha K. Swartz, PhD, RN, CPNP (Co-chair, NAPNAP)

xiv

INTRODUCTION

Pediatric nursing is the protection, promotion, and optimization of health and abilities for children of newborn age through young adulthood. Utilizing a family-centered care approach, pediatric nursing includes the prevention of illness and injury, the alleviation of suffering through the diagnosis and treatment of the child's response, and advocacy in the care of children and families.

Pediatric Nursing: Scope and Standards of Practice is intended to be used in conjunction with *Nursing: Scope and Standards of Practice* (ANA, 2004), *Nursing's Social Policy Statement* (ANA, 2003), *Code of Ethics for Nurses with Interpretive Statements* (ANA, 2001), *Domains and Core Competencies of Nurse Practitioner Practice* (National Organization of Nurse Practitioner Faculties, 2006a), and other documents that outline the values, beliefs, and practice patterns of pediatric nurses. *Pediatric Nursing: Scope and Standards of Practice* reflects and guides the practice of nurses in generalist and advanced practice roles who provide clinical care to children and their families. It may also provide useful information to families and stakeholders such as administrators, educators, policy makers, and others invested in accessing, delivering, and financing health care. Additionally, the document will provide guidance in evaluating the effectiveness and appropriateness of healthcare delivery in pediatric settings.

The National Association of Pediatric Nurse Practitioners (NAPNAP) broadly defines the pediatric population as including all children from birth through 21 years of age, and in specific situations to individuals older than 21 years until appropriate transition to adult health care is successful (NAPNAP, 2002a). There are a growing number of adolescents and young adults with special healthcare needs, chronic conditions, and disabilities who need transition care from pediatric to adult healthcare settings (Betz, 2003, 2004a, & 2004b). With an extensive knowledge base regarding developmental issues and concerns of adolescents and young adults, pediatric nurses are qualified to assist youth during the transition phase. To create an exclusive upper age limit for pediatric patients may unnecessarily create barriers and limit access to health care for this population.

Pediatric Nursing: Scope of Practice 1

Function of the Scope of Practice Statement

A scope of practice statement describes the *who, what, where, when, why,* and *how* of nursing practice. Each of these questions must be sufficiently answered to provide a complete picture of the practice, its boundaries, and membership. The depth and breadth in which individual nurses engage in the total scope of nursing practice is dependent upon education, certification, individual states' nursing rules and regulations, experience, role, and the population served.

Definition and Function of Standards

Standards are authoritative statements in which the nursing profession describes the responsibilities for which its practitioners are accountable. Consequently, standards reflect the values and priorities of the profession. Standards provide direction for professional nursing practice and a framework for the evaluation of practice. Written in measurable terms, standards also define the nursing profession's accountability to the public and the practice outcomes for which nurses are responsible.

Development of Standards

Standards of professional nursing practice may pertain to general or specialty practice. Each professional nursing organization has a responsibility to its membership and the public it serves to develop standards of practice. This publication is the result of a joint collaboration between the National Association of Pediatric Nurse Practitioners (NAPNAP) and the Society of Pediatric Nurses (SPN). It sets forth standards of pediatric nursing practice and applies them to all nurses engaged in the care of children and their families across care settings. It is based on the original *Scope and Standards of Pediatric Nursing Practice* (ANA & SPN, 2003), *Scope and Standards of Practice: Pediatric Nurse Practitioner (PNP)* (NAPNAP, 2004b) and *Nursing: Scope and Standards of Practice* (ANA, 2004). This document describes aspects of competent nursing care and professional performance which are measurable, can be evaluated, and are common to nurses engaged in the care of children and their families based on their generalist or advanced practice role.

2   *Pediatric Nursing: Scope and Standards of Practice*

Assumptions

Pediatric Nursing: Scope and Standards of Practice focuses primarily on the processes of providing pediatric nursing care at the generalist and advanced practice levels, and the performance of professional role activities. These standards apply to all nurses involved in the care of children and their families, and they are applicable despite the extensive variability among practice settings. Recognizing the link between the professional work environment and the pediatric nurse's ability to deliver care, employers must provide an environment supportive of nursing practice.

The first major assumption underlying this document is that nursing care is individualized to meet a particular child's or family's unique needs and situation, while focusing on individual, cultural, ethnic, and religious values and beliefs. This includes respect for the goals and preferences of the child and family in developing and implementing a plan of care. Given that one of the nurse's primary responsibilities is need-based patient education, pediatric nurses provide children and their families with individualized information, which empowers children and their families to make informed decisions regarding their health care, including health promotion, prevention of disease, and attainment of a peaceful death.

A second major assumption is that the pediatric nurse establishes a partnership with the child, family, and other healthcare providers. In this partnership, the nurse works collaboratively to coordinate care provided to the child and family. The degree of participation by the child and family will vary based upon preference and ability, and in the case of the child, upon age, developmental abilities, and cognitive understanding of the plan of care.

Organizing Principles

According to *Nursing's Social Policy Statement* (ANA 2003), the recipients of nursing care are individuals, groups, families, communities, and populations. *Pediatric Nursing: Scope and Standards of Practice* uses the terms "client," "patient," "child," and "family" to indicate the person(s) for whom the nurse is providing health care. Care is provided to assist the child or family, sick or well, in performance of those activities contributing to health or its recovery (or to peaceful death), and a return to

Pediatric Nursing: Scope of Practice   3

independence that the child or family would perform unaided if they had the necessary skills, strength, will or knowledge (Alexander et al., 1998; Henderson, 1964).

Consideration of the cultural, racial, ethnic, social, economic, and developmental aspects of the child and family is essential to the provision of nursing services and for developing a plan of care. Precise descriptions of children's health status require viewing children and youth within the context of their environment and development continuum (World Health Organization [WHO] 2007). The *International Classification of Functioning, Disability and Health—Children and Youth Version (ICF–CY)*, which applies classification codes to hundreds of bodily functions and structures, activities, and participation, and various environmental factors that restrict or allow young people to function in an array of everyday activities, enables the accurate and constructive description of children's health (WHO, 2007). Additionally, clients with developmental disabilities are present in all communities and care settings, remaining a vulnerable population. Whatever their age, they and their families need assurance of safe and effective nursing care (Nehring et al. , 2004).

Pediatric Nursing: Scope and Standards of Practice addresses the scope of practice for pediatric nursing which applies to all registered nurses engaged in the nursing care of children and their families, regardless of clinical specialty, practice setting, or educational preparation. Standards that further define the responsibilities of nurses working with children and families in advanced practice roles are also articulated in this document.

Pediatric Nursing: Scope and Standards of Practice provides 16 standards that are categorized as standards of practice and standards of professional performance:

Standards of Practice
1. Assessment
2. Diagnosis
3. Outcomes Identification
4. Planning
5. Implementation

4   *Pediatric Nursing: Scope and Standards of Practice*

5a. Coordination of Care and Case Management

5b. Health Teaching and Health Promotion, Restoration, and Maintenance

5c. Consultation

5d. Prescriptive Authority and Treatment

5e. Referral

6. Evaluation

Standards of Professional Performance

7. Quality of Practice

8. Professional Practice Evaluation

9. Education

10. Collegiality

11. Ethics

12. Collaboration

13. Research, Evidence-Based Practice, and Clinical Scholarship

14. Resource Utilization

15. Leadership

16. Advocacy

Each category of standards is described below:

Standards of Practice

The six standards of practice describe a competent level of nursing care, as demonstrated by the nursing process, including assessment, diagnosis, outcome identification, planning, implementation, and evaluation. The nursing process encompasses all significant actions taken by nurses in providing care to all patients and families, and it forms the foundation for clinical decision-making and the integration of best research evidence with clinical expertise and patient values (Sackett, Straus, Richardson, Rosenberg, & Haynes 2000). Several themes are common to all areas of nursing practice and reflect nursing responsibilities for all

Pediatric Nursing: Scope of Practice 5

The content in this appendix is not current and is of historical significance only.

children and their families. These themes merit additional attention and include:

- Providing age-appropriate and culturally and ethnically sensitive care
- Maintaining a safe environment
- Educating children and their families about health practices and treatment modalities
- Providing care that is family-centered as well as efficient, respectful of time, and fiscally responsible
- Ensuring continuity of care
- Coordinating care across settings and among caregivers
- Managing and protecting information
- Communicating effectively inter-professionally and within nursing, as well as in nurse–child–parent interactions
- Ensuring the implementation of evidence-based clinical findings in the practice setting

These themes will be reflected in the measurement criteria associated with various standards in this document, although the wording may be different. They are highlighted here because they are fundamental to many of the standards, and because they have emerged as being consistently and significantly influential in nursing practice today.

Standards of Professional Performance

The ten standards of professional performance describe a competent level of behavior in the professional role, including activities related to quality of care, performance appraisal, outcomes measurement, education, collegiality, ethics, collaboration, research and clinical scholarship, resource utilization, leadership, professional accountability, and advocacy. Within these standards, the advanced practice nurse is expected to be accountable for several other responsibilities that comprise the hallmarks of the profession as well as the advanced practice role. These activities include serving in leadership positions within professional organizations, serving as a role model or mentor to other pediatric nurses, participating in family-centered research, and using evidence-

6   *Pediatric Nursing: Scope and Standards of Practice*

based practice processes to ensure a practice based on evidence. All nurses are expected to engage in professional role activities appropriate to their education, position, and practice setting. Ultimately, nurses are accountable to themselves, patients, and peers for their professional actions.

Measurement Criteria

Pediatric Nursing: Scope and Standards of Practice includes criteria that allow the standards to be measured. These criteria include key indicators of competent practice. To achieve the standards of practice, all criteria must be met, with additional criteria for the advanced practice nurse. Standards should remain stable over time, as they reflect the philosophical values of the profession. However, criteria may be revised to incorporate advancements in scientific knowledge and clinical practice, consultations with other healthcare professionals, and individualized family needs. Criteria must also remain consistent with current nursing practice, education, and research.

Throughout this document, terms such as "appropriate," "pertinent," and "realistic" are used. This document cannot account for all possible scenarios that the pediatric nurse might encounter in clinical practice. The pediatric nurse will need to exercise judgment based on education and experience in determining what is appropriate, pertinent, or realistic. Further direction may be available from documents such as guidelines for practice or agency standards, policies, procedures, protocols, and literature reviews.

Guidelines

Guidelines describe a process of patient care management that has the potential for improving the quality of clinical and consumer decision-making. As systematically developed statements based on available scientific evidence, clinical expertise, and expert opinion, guidelines address the care of specific patient populations or phenomena, whereas standards provide a broad framework for practice. Many practice guidelines have been developed by professional organizations that are applicable to the pediatric population. Guidelines may be used to provide direction for clinical practice policies, procedures, and protocols.

Pediatric Nursing: Scope of Practice 7

Appendix B. Pediatric Nursing: Scope and Standards of Practice (2008)

Summary

Pediatric Nursing: Scope and Standards of Practice delineates the professional responsibilities of registered (including advanced practice) nurses engaged in clinical practice related to children and their families, regardless of setting. *Pediatric Nursing: Scope and Standards of Practice* and other nursing practice guidelines serve as a basis for:

- Quality improvement systems
- Data system development
- Regulatory systems
- Healthcare reimbursement and financing methodologies
- Development and evaluation of nursing service delivery systems and organizational structures
- Certification activities
- Job descriptions and performance appraisals
- Agency policies, procedures, and protocols
- Educational offerings
- Research activities
- Consistency in care
- Professional development
- Global health

In order to best serve the public and the nursing profession, pediatric nurses must continue to contribute to the development of standards of practice and evidence-based practice guidelines. Nursing must examine how standards and practice guidelines can be disseminated and used more effectively to enhance and promote the quality of clinical practice. In addition, standards and practice guidelines must be evaluated on an ongoing basis, with revisions made as necessary. The dynamic nature of the healthcare environment and the growing body of nursing research provide both the impetus and the opportunity for nursing to ensure competent clinical practice and to promote ongoing professional development that enhances the quality of pediatric nursing care.

SCOPE OF PEDIATRIC NURSING PRACTICE

The scope of practice and roles of the pediatric nurse are diverse and dynamic. The intention of this document is to identify some of the issues and trends that define current roles and to highlight the variety of pediatric nursing roles that have evolved to meet the ever-changing healthcare needs of children and their families in a variety of settings. The document is not intended to restrict role development, but rather to clarify the scope and foundation of general as well as advanced practice pediatric nursing and to distinguish between these areas of practice.

Practice Context

There are approximately 73 million children and adolescents in the United States, accounting for one-fourth of the nation's population (U.S. Department of Health and Human Services, 2005). Approximately 20% of children experience special healthcare needs, chronic illness, or disability. The most prevalent chronic conditions among children are asthma (affecting 12% of children), learning disabilities (affecting 8%) and attention-deficit hyperactivity disorder (affecting 7%).

For children and adolescents who do not experience a chronic illness or condition, major threats to health include accidents, violence, substance abuse, and sexually transmitted illnesses. Injuries are the leading cause of death among those 1 to 24 years of age, and over 50% of injuries are related to motor vehicle collisions (U.S. Department of Health and Human Services, 2002).

Children, families, and all citizens are significantly affected by the growing problem of youth violence. According to an integrative review (Gance-Cleveland, 2001), youths are three times more likely than adults to be victims of a violent crime, and homicide is the second leading cause of death among youths age 15–24 years. It is estimated that 270,000 guns are taken to school each day in the United States, while firearms in the home also provide a risk for unintentional injury. Overall, the threat of terrorism and bioterrorism places further stress and strain on the ability of children and their families to cope with uncertainty.

In the United States, minorities and the poor experience disparities in access to health care, health-related quality of life, and illness and death.

Pediatric Nursing: Scope of Practice 9

A recent analysis by the Children's Defense Fund (CDF) of data from the National Health Interview Survey revealed significant racial and ethnic differences of the effects of healthcare coverage and income on outcomes (CDF, 2006). Among the findings by the CDF are:

- Latino children are almost three times as likely and African–American children are almost twice as likely as Caucasian children to be uninsured;

- among the uninsured, African–American children are 60% more likely than Caucasian children to have an unmet healthcare need; and

- similar percentages of African–American and Caucasian low-income children have gone two or more years without receiving dental care and have experienced limitations due to a chronic illness or disability.

The findings of the CDF further indicate that among children, disparities persist in the rates of infant mortality, immunizations, asthma, lead poisoning, and obesity. These are conditions that may impact many aspects of a child's health and development and can have lasting effects throughout adolescence and into adulthood. Because childhood is a time of physical, social, intellectual, and emotional growth, pediatric nursing practice must be aimed at the prevention, early identification, and intervention for health problems that may extend to adulthood. To reduce healthcare disparities, pediatric nurses advocate for and provide quality health care. Additionally, they work with the community and policy makers to foster awareness of child health disparities, and they may work with other clinicians and public health officials in coalitions to identify resources, and implement and evaluate programs of health care.

To further explore the effect of recent governmental programs on children's access to health care, a pediatric nurse practitioner (PNP) headed an evaluative study of the State Child Health Insurance Program (SCHIP), published in *Pediatrics* (Duderstadt, Hughes, Soobader & Newacheck, 2006). Like the CDF, Duderstadt and colleagues also analyzed data comparing the 1997 and 2003 National Health Interview Survey. Findings revealed that children in the SCHIP target income group experienced the largest reduction in rates of uninsurance, and the percentage of children without a usual source of care or a primary care provider was also reduced. However, the implementation of the SCHIP program led to no significant changes in the level of reported unmet needs, volume of provider visits, receipt of well-child care, and dental care. Thus, while the SCHIP program has increased the rates of Medicaid enrollment for children in eligible families, healthcare disparities persist. Pediatric nurses are key to advocating for families, making policy recommendations, and evaluating the effects of such programs through research and education.

Quality and Outcome Guidelines for Nursing of Children and Families

Beginning in 2001, the Expert Panel on Children and Families of the American Academy of Nursing initiated a collaborative process to identify the key standards of excellence in the nursing of children and families (Craft-Rosenberg & Krajicek, 2006). These guidelines were developed by a coalition of pediatric and family nurses representing 12 professional organizations, including SPN and NAPNAP. The 18 guidelines of this "paradigm of excellence" provide a template for clinicians, educators, researchers, and policy makers to promote, evaluate, and improve the quality of health care that is provided to children and families (Table 1).

The recently published text *Nursing Excellence for Children and Families* devotes a chapter to each of the guidelines, with each chapter presenting a review and analysis of the evidence pertaining to the guideline as well as implications for practice (Craft-Rosenberg & Krajicek, 2006). Clinicians may apply the guidelines to evaluate and change nursing care in the clinical setting. They may also be used by educators for curriculum revision and by researchers as a framework for testing interventions to evaluate effectiveness and outcomes. A consumer version of the guidelines has also been developed so that patients and families may evaluate the quality of care received.

Healthcare Home

The concept *healthcare home* or *medical home* provides a framework to improve access to care and eliminate disparities in health (including dental) care for children and families through effective care coordination and case management (Cowell & Swartwout, 2006). NAPNAP advocates for a pediatric healthcare home that is "accessible, comprehensive, coordinated, culturally sensitive and focused on the overall well-being

Pediatric Nursing: Scope of Practice 11

T A B L E 1 Healthcare Quality and Outcome Guidelines

1. Children and youth have an identified healthcare home.
2. The families of children and youth are partners in decisions, planning, and delivery of care.
3. Family values, beliefs, and preferences are part of care.
4. Family strengths and main concerns are obvious in the care of children and youth.
5. Children, youth, and families will have accessible health care.
6. Pregnant women will have accessible health care.
7. Family needs are identified and services are offered.
8. Children, youth, and families are directed to community services when needed.
9. Children, youth, and families receive care that promotes and maintains health and prevents disease.
10. Pregnant women, children, youth, and families have access to genetic testing and advice.
11. Children and youth receive care that is physically and emotionally safe.
12. Children's, youth's, and families' privacy and rights are protected.
13. Children and youth who are very ill receive the full range of needed services.
14. Children and youth with disabilities and/or special healthcare needs receive the full range of services.
15. Children, youth, and families receive comfort care.
16. Children's, youths', and families' health and risky behaviors and problems are identified and addressed.
17. Children, youth, and families receive care that supports development.
18. Children, youth, and families are fully informed of the outcomes of care.

From Craft-Rosenberg, M. & Krajicek, M. (2006). *Nursing excellence for children and families*. New York, NY: Springer Publishing Co.

of the child within the family" (NAPNAP, 2002b). NAPNAP further asserts that all children should have access to comprehensive health care by their pediatric healthcare professional of choice, and that all healthcare providers, including pediatricians, pediatric subspecialists, pediatric nurse practitioners, nurses, and clinical nurse specialists, should have a collaborative role in the provision of such care. Such care should be available without barriers to service resulting from financial or insurance restrictions, lack of available providers, or other difficulties (NAPNAP, 2007).

While *healthcare home* or *medical home* is a relatively new label, the elements of such care can historically be traced back to public health

12   ***Pediatric Nursing: Scope and Standards of Practice***

nursing and the community mental health movement which provided guidelines for providing care to the underserved (APHA, 1955; Caplan, 1961; Pridham, 1993). Nursing has continued to be a driving force in the development of innovative models for providing high quality health care including school-based health centers (SBHCs) and community health centers. Because nurses interact with consumers at multiple entry points in the healthcare system, they play a key role in implementing the healthcare home concept and assuring that care is accessible, comprehensive, continuous, and culturally competent. According to Cowell & Swartwout (2006), nursing care excellence in implementing the healthcare home concept is achieved by:

- supporting the delivery of care via interdisciplinary teams;
- creating effective communication and partnerships with each family;
- enabling a central location for healthcare records;
- involving family members and individualizing care;
- being an expert at knowing community resources;
- being an expert on state and federal policies, regulations, and programs;
- implementing a quality monitoring system;
- promoting and monitoring preventive care;
- providing comprehensive primary care;
- providing creative solutions for those who are uninsured;
- providing support during periods of transition;
- working with families with special needs;
- assisting families in becoming independent, informed consumers of health care; and
- generating nursing research related to the healthcare home concept.

Family-Centered Care and Management Styles

Family-Centered Care is a philosophy of care that acknowledges the importance of family partnerships in nursing care whereby the family is an active partner or collaborator in the process, not a passive recipient of the professional's expertise (Deatrick, 2006). With an increase in

Pediatric Nursing: Scope of Practice   13

the number of single-parent and blended families, traditional definitions of family that are grounded in biological ties are no longer useful. Shelton and Stepanek (1994) maintain that the first step in providing Family-Centered Care is to understand how a family defines itself and who the child considers as family members.

The Family-Centered Care model recognizes the family as the constant in the child's life and central in the child's plan of care. Eight elements of Family-Centered Care have been defined, each serving to reinforce, facilitate, and complement the implementation of the others (see Table 2). These elements recognize each family's uniqueness, acknowledge the influence of the family as a constant in the child's life, and emphasize the importance of providing health care which reflects the value of collaboration between the child, family, and the healthcare team. Family-Centered Care is based upon the premise that a positive adjustment to a child's level of health and well-being requires the involvement of the whole family. *Family-Centered Care: Putting it into Action—The SPN/ANA Guide to Family-Centered Care* further expands upon these elements and provides evidence-based practice recommendations that more fully describe this model (Lewandowski & Tesler, 2003).

In order to build partnerships with families, nurses and healthcare providers need standardized guidelines and descriptions of family coping styles in order to individualize their approaches to families. The Family Management Style (FMS) framework was developed over a 20-year period through reviews of qualitative research and concept development. Five family management styles or patterns describing how families define and manage illness-related demands and the resulting consequences for family life have emerged: thriving, accommodating, enduring, struggling, and floundering (Deatrick & Knafl, 1990; Knafl, Breitmayer, Gallo & Zoeller 1996; Knafl & Deatrick 2002). The styles represent the continuum of difficulties that families experience when managing a child's illness and also provide a basis for individualized care planning.

Evidence-based Practice

There is concern among healthcare organizations, federal agencies, and the public regarding the large time gap between the publication of

14   *Pediatric Nursing: Scope and Standards of Practice*

T A B L E 2 Key Elements of Family-Centered Care

Element 1: The Family at the Center

Incorporate into policy and practice the recognition that family is the constant in a child's life, while the service systems and support personnel within those systems fluctuate and that the illness or injury of a child affects all members of the family.

Element 2: Family–Professional Collaboration

Facilitate family-professional collaboration at all levels of hospital, home, and community care for:

- Care of an individual child;
- Program development, implementation, evaluation and evolution;
- Policy formation.

Element 3: Family-Professional Communication

Exchange complete and unbiased information between families and professionals in a supportive manner at all times.

Element 4: Cultural Diversity of the Family

Incorporate into policy and practice the recognition and of honoring of cultural diversity, strengths, and individuality within and across all families, including ethnic,racial, spiritual, social, economic, educational, and geographic diversity.

Element 5: Coping Differences and Supports

Recognize and respect different methods of coping and implement comprehensive policies and programs that provide families with the developmental, educational, emotional, spiritual, environmental, and financial supports needed to meet their diverse needs.

Element 6: Family-Centered Peer Support

Encourage and facilitate family-to-family support networking.

Element 7: Specialized Service and Support Systems

Ensure that hospital, home, and community service and support systems for children needing specialized health and developmental care and their families are flexible, accessible, and comprehensive in responding to diverse family-identified needs.

Element 8: Holistic Perspective of Family-Centered Care

Appreciate families as families and children as children, recognizing that they possess a wide range of strengths, concerns emotions and aspirations beyond their need for specialized health and developmental services and support.

From Lewandowski, L. & Tesler, M. (2003). *Family-Centered Care: Putting it Into Action – The SPN/ANA Guide to Family-Centered Care.* Washington, DC: Nursebooks.org.

Pediatric Nursing: Scope of Practice   **15**

Appendix B. Pediatric Nursing: Scope and Standards of Practice (2008)

research findings and the translation of findings into practice to improve patient care. Furthermore, the findings reported by the Institute of Medicine (2001) in *Crossing the Quality Chasm: A New Health System for the 21st Century* have challenged all healthcare professionals to deliver care that is based upon the best scientific evidence available. Evidence-based practice (EBP) has been defined as "the integration of best research evidence with clinical expertise and patient values" (Sackett, Straus, Richardson, Rosenberg & Haynes, 2000). In nursing, several evidence-based nursing centers have been developed at leading universities (Brady & Lewin, 2007).

Increasingly, clinical practice guidelines are being developed by professional organizations or expert panels that promote the translation of evidence-based findings into nursing care (Melnyk & Fineout-Overholt, 2005). One such example is the *Healthy Eating and Activity Together (HEAT^SM) Clinical Practice Guideline: Identifying and Preventing Overweight in Childhood*, published by NAPNAP (2006b), which is aimed at the prevention of overweight and obesity in children. A key component of this guideline is the inclusion of culturally appropriate strategies for groups most at risk for childhood overweight (Hispanics, African–Americans, and Native Americans).

Similarly, NAPNAP has also developed the national program *KySS^SM: Keep Your Children/Yourself Safe and Secure*, and a supporting *The KySS^SM Guide to Child and Adolescent Mental Health Screening, Early Intervention and Health Promotion* (Melnyk & Moldenhauer, 2006) which is geared toward the prevention and subsequent decrease of psychosocial morbidities in children and teenagers. The program emphasizes educational–behavioral interventions to teach children, youth, and their parents all aspects of physical and emotional safety, and to build self-esteem, and to strengthen other developmental assets such as positive coping and problem-solving skills.

Pediatric nurses acknowledge the need for evidence-based practice in the clinical setting and recognize that continuing research, including research involving children, will be required to gather that evidence. Pediatric nurses advocate for research where minimal risk to the child is involved and potential benefits outweigh risks. Pediatric nurses promote research that is conducted in a respectful, ethical manner in the hope that findings will benefit the children involved in the studies and the future care of children (NAPNAP, 2004a; SPN, 2004).

16   *Pediatric Nursing: Scope and Standards of Practice*

Differentiated Areas of Pediatric Nursing Practice

Pediatric nurses are licensed registered nurses who provide health care to children through either a generalist or advanced practice role. These areas of practice are described below.

Pediatric Nurse: Generalist

The pediatric nurse who practices as a *generalist* is a licensed registered nurse who has demonstrated clinical skills and knowledge within the specialty. Many nurses who contribute to the care of children and their families are also responsible for adhering to the specialty practice standards as designated by the profession.

In 1998, SPN completed a project funded by the Health Resources and Services Administration (HRSA) Maternal and Child Bureau that identified standards for pediatric pre-licensure and early professional development (Woodring & Pridham, 1998). While these concepts and competencies apply to the education of the beginning practitioner, they offer a unique description of the elements of pediatric nursing including:

- the unique anatomical, physiological, and developmental differences among neonates, infants, children, adolescents, and young adults in transition;

- care of children in the context of their families;

- sensitivity to cultural issues, especially those related to how the family and healthcare providers tend to children's healthcare needs;

- effective communication with children, families, other healthcare providers, and appropriate educational agency staff;

- safety assurance and injury prevention for children and their families;

- promotion of children's health in the context of their families;

- assessment of the unique growth and development needs of children who have chronic conditions, and of their families;

- exceptional needs of children with episodic injuries or illnesses;

- economic, social, and political influences outside the family that have an impact on children's health and development and family functioning; and

- ethical, moral, and legal dilemmas involving children, families, and healthcare professionals.

Pediatric Nursing: Scope of Practice   17

Advanced Practice Pediatric Nurse

Advanced practice registered nurses (APRNs) are registered nurses (RNs) who have acquired advanced education (either a master's or doctoral degree) and have developed specialized clinical knowledge and skills to provide health care. They build upon the practice of RNs by demonstrating a greater depth and breadth of knowledge, a strong ability to synthesize data and employ critical thinking, increased complexity of skills and interventions, and significant role autonomy (ANA, 2004). The APRN role combines both specialization and expansion through in-depth study of the research-based, theoretical, and clinical practice issues unique to the specialty population.

In pediatric nursing, the predominant advanced practice roles are the pediatric clinical nurse specialist (PCNS), the primary care pediatric nurse practitioner (PNP-PC), the acute care pediatric nurse practitioner (PNP-AC), and the neonatal nurse practitioner (NNP). The advanced practice pediatric nurse holds a minimum of a master's degree in pediatric nursing, has attained certification in the advanced practice role, and holds the appropriate credentials as determined by the state Board of Nursing. The pediatric APRN provides care in an expanded role that incorporates comprehensive assessment skills, diagnostic ability, critical thinking, independent decision-making, collaborative management of health and illness problems, leadership within complex systems, and the ability to critically analyze and translate research findings into practice. APRNs in other clinical settings, such as family practice, nurse midwifery, and nurse anesthesia, are also expected to incorporate advanced knowledge of pediatric concepts into their clinical practice to the extent that their client populations may include pediatric patients and their families.

The advanced practice pediatric nursing roles are differentiated from one another by virtue of their unique blend of nursing knowledge, science, and practice settings. The following descriptions further illustrate the advanced practice roles which require knowledge specialization and clinical expertise in the care of children and their families:

Pediatric Clinical Nurse Specialist (PCNS)

The PCNS is an APRN prepared as a clinical expert in the specialty of pediatric nursing and who, in addition to providing direct patient care, serves as a leader in education, research, quality improvement, outcome monitoring, and consultation with other nurses, health team members,

18   *Pediatric Nursing: Scope and Standards of Practice*

and the community. Clinical nurse specialists are prepared at the master's or doctoral level. CNSs are generally employed and paid by a healthcare institution, or they may work independently in private or collaborative practice. The National Association of Clinical Nurse Specialists (NACNS) has published a position statement on CNS education and practice in which they identify core CNS competencies and the corresponding core areas of knowledge that should be included in CNS graduate programs (NACNS 2004). The core areas of knowledge are expanded from the core areas identified in the American Association of Colleges of Nursing's (AACN) *Essentials of Master's Education for Advance Practice Nursing* (1996) document and include theoretical foundations, inquiry skills, empirical and practical knowledge that focus on phenomena of concern, nursing therapeutics, evaluation methodologies, and systems thinking.

Pediatric Nurse Practitioner (PNP)

The PNP provides comprehensive health care to children from birth through young adulthood by assessment, diagnosis, management, and evaluation of care. In accordance with state licensure and regulatory mechanisms, PNPs provide a wide range of pediatric healthcare services in a variety of primary and specialty healthcare settings, with a strong emphasis on health promotion, injury and disease prevention, and management and coping with chronic illness. The PNP may consult with other members of the healthcare team, coordinate care, and make referrals to other healthcare providers. Additionally, the PNP may function as a consultant in areas of expertise to colleagues in health professions and other disciplines. The PNP assumes accountability for professional actions and incorporates risk management strategies into clinical practice. Today, PNPs practice not only in primary care but also in acute and specialty care settings. While the types of settings have expanded, the fundamental aspects and essential components of the PNP remain consistent across settings. There are now two broad categories of PNPs: those who practice predominantly in primary care settings and those who practice in acute care settings.

Historically, PNPs have practiced predominantly in primary care settings in which the emphasis is on providing health care that is accessible, comprehensive in scope, and coordinated with specialty practices and community resources in order to maximize continuity. Certification

Pediatric Nursing: Scope of Practice   **19**

as a PNP, with an emphasis on primary care, is offered by both the Pediatric Nursing Certification Board (PNCB) and the American Nurses Credentialing Center (ANCC) and is required for recognition in most states.

The acute care PNP provides cost-effective, quality care for acutely, critically, and chronically ill children who may be experiencing life-threatening illnesses and organ dysfunction or failure. Similar to the primary care PNP, direct patient care management by the acute care PNP within a collaborative practice model includes performing in-depth physical assessments, ordering and interpreting results of laboratory and diagnostic tests, ordering medications, and performing therapeutic procedures in a variety of contexts which may include inpatient and outpatient hospital units, emergency departments, and home care settings. The foundation of advanced practice nursing also provides general role expectations for the acute care PNP which include expertise in patient care that is based on clinical evidence and theory, progressive leadership, and involvement in education and research.

The role of the acute care PNP began to evolve in the late 1990s, as nurse practitioner practice expanded into critical care units, specialty practice sites, and emergency departments. The expansion of the role was also in keeping with recommendations of the Institute of Medicine, which called for a greater commitment to interdisciplinary care (2001). The increased demand for PNPs with knowledge and skills necessary for acute care practice led to progressive changes in the education of PNPs for this role. In 2004, NAPNAP developed a position statement for the acute care PNP (NAPNAP, 2005a). Similarly, the National Panel for Acute Care Nurse Practitioner Competencies, in collaboration with the Association of Faculties of PNP Programs (AFPNP), developed a set of core competencies for PNPs in acute care (2004). These competencies now provide the basis for curriculum development, evaluation, and certification. The PNCB offered the first certification examination for the acute care PNP in January 2005 to those who met the standards of review by the PNCB, based on the competencies. Currently, graduation from an acute care PNP program is required to sit for the PNCB acute care PNP examination. As with other nursing roles, the requirements for entry into practice and for recognition of the acute care PNP role vary from state to state. As of this writing, the majority of states (31) require that acute care PNPs take a

20   *Pediatric Nursing: Scope and Standards of Practice*

pediatric acute care certification examination in order to be fully licensed by the state (Percy & Sperhac, 2007).

Neonatal Nurse Practitioner (NNP)

NNPs provide healthcare services to high-risk infants in neonatal intensive care units (NICUs), well baby nurseries, and in follow-up clinics (for children 2 years of age and younger). The NNP services include providing diagnosis and management of neonatal diseases, health promotion, and follow-up care of high-risk babies. NNP competencies have also been developed by the National Association of Neonatal Nurses (NANN) to reflect the educational standards for neonatal nurse practitioner programs (NANN, 2002). The standards are based on a foundation of the broad standards for advanced nursing practice (American Association of Colleges of Nursing 1996) and the evaluation criteria for nurse practitioner programs.

All nurse practitioners and clinical nurse specialists function according to their state Nurse Practice Act and in accordance with individual state laws and regulations. States vary in their regulations, including the granting of prescriptive privileges, and specific state requirements must be recognized and met. In some states, current impediments to the full use of advanced practice nurses include:

(1) legal barriers such as laws that require physician supervision or limit a nurse's prescriptive authority,

(2) financial barriers that prevent public and private payers from reimbursing advanced practice nurses, and

(3) professional barriers.

As Safriet (1992) has stated, "Advanced practice nurses have demonstrated repeatedly that they can provide cost-effective, high quality primary care for many of the neediest members of society, but their role has been severely limited by restrictions on their scope of practice, prescriptive authority, and eligibility for reimbursement" (p. 417). Fortunately, healthcare regulatory organizations now acknowledge that it is not reasonable to expect each health profession to have a completely unique scope of practice, and that there is considerable overlap among the abilities and skill sets of each discipline (Association of Social Work Boards et al, 2007). Scope of practice changes

Pediatric Nursing: Scope of Practice   21

Appendix B. Pediatric Nursing: Scope and Standards of Practice (2008)

should reflect the evolution of the abilities of practitioners within a healthcare discipline to provide care in a safe and effective manner, in order to better protect the public and enhance consumer access to quality health care.

Settings for Pediatric Nursing Practice

Inpatient and Acute Care Settings

Practice settings for pediatric nursing are multiple and varied. Free-standing children's hospitals, which are solely dedicated to providing acute care and rehabilitation services to the pediatric population, represent just 1% of all hospitals, but account for 39% of all admissions, 49% of inpatient days, and 59% of hospital costs (National Association of Children's Hospitals and Related Institutions, 2001). There are other facilities (e.g., pediatric and adolescent units, pediatric and neonatal intensive care units) where pediatric specialty services are provided within a multi-focused acute care setting. Children's hospitals and major teaching hospitals together treat 98% of all children requiring heart or lung transplants, 88% of all children with cancer needing in-patient care, and 76% of all children hospitalized with cystic fibrosis (National Association of Children's Hospitals and Related Institutions, 2001). In addition, children's hospitals are key providers for the 35% of children who are either uninsured or dependent on Medicaid and other public sources for payment of health care.

Perioperative and Surgical Settings

The pediatric surgical environment creates an additional setting for pediatric nursing. Pediatric surgical nursing involves care for children throughout the surgical experience, including pre-operative preparation and teaching, intra-operative care in both inpatient and out-patient settings, and post-operative care for major surgery, minimally invasive surgery, innovative therapies, fetal surgery, pediatric solid organ transplantation, surgery for congenital anomalies, and more. Perioperative nurses provide direct patient care, coordinate the multi-disciplinary surgical care team, and provide emotional and psycho-social support to the family and child. The American Pediatric Surgical Nurses Association (APSNA) is the specialty organization for those pediatric nurses involved in perioperative nursing.

Hospice and Palliative Care Settings

In the United States, it is estimated that 53,000 children from newborns through 19 years of age die each year, with 75–85% of children dying in the hospital—many in the intensive care setting (Field & Behrman, 2003). Less than 1% of these children die in a pediatric hospice setting.

Palliative care, which can take place in the hospital or home setting, focuses on enhancing the quality of remaining life by assisting the child and family to meet the goals they have set. It is not meant to hasten or postpone death but coexists with curative measures. Care can change as the child advances through the disease process and as death approaches. Palliative care can give dignity to life and allows death to happen in a manner that is meaningful for the family. When families are faced with complex medical or life decisions regarding the care of their child, such as whether to continue or withhold treatment, the pediatric palliative nurse can facilitate patient–family communication, provide specific clinical information, and assist with the palliative care plan.

Hospice care is care provided at the end of life where the disease has been deemed either incurable or terminal with a life expectancy of six months or less. The focus is non-curative treatment with aggressive management of symptoms aimed at improving the quality of life at the end of life and facilitating bereavement once death has occurred. The pediatric hospice nurse assists the family through the dying and bereavement process.

Ambulatory Care Settings

Ambulatory care settings offer children and their families ongoing contact with healthcare professionals. Due to long-term, ongoing contact with the family, the nurse in this setting has an opportunity to develop a mutually gratifying and therapeutic relationship with the child and family. This long-term relationship can provide a more complete picture of the child's general well-being and ability to achieve developmental milestones. Illness prevention and health promotion activities are the core interventions of the nurse and the healthcare team. For children coping with a chronic condition, the healthcare team also focuses on maintaining optimum levels of health for the child.

The nurse practicing in a specialty pediatric clinic collaborates with a multidisciplinary team to meet the challenges of patients with a

Pediatric Nursing: Scope of Practice   **23**

chronic or terminal illness. Quality health care for these children often requires significant case coordination so that the care provided is accessible, comprehensive, continuous, and efficient. Throughout the care process, the nurse serves as a vital link in the communication between health team members and the family.

Community Health and School Settings

Community health settings provide the pediatric nurse an opportunity to positively affect large populations of children and families through community health organizations, schools, and city and state departments of health. Many community health programs are aimed at prevention, education, and provision of programs (such as immunizations and screening). Pediatric nurses practicing in home health care address the environmental, social, and personal factors affecting health and may provide care that cannot be offered by family or friends on a consistent basis. The focus of home health care is on preventing admission to an acute care setting, providing assistance to families, and providing direct treatment in the home.

Pediatric nurses working in schools may be employed by a local school system (either public or private), or by a county, city, or state governmental agency. The National Association of School Nurses (NASN) developed a resolution paper on the need for access to school nurses and a position statement outlining the need for school nurses in caring for chronically ill children (NASN, 2003, 2006). The school nurse is often responsible for meeting the needs of children in more than one school and ideally works with an aide, health associate, and other unlicensed assistive personnel who are responsible for monitoring day-to-day school health problems. The school nurse is responsible for overall management and delegation of activities to the aides and for evaluating the appropriateness of interventions provided to ailing children.

School nursing is a specialized practice of professional nursing that advances the well-being, academic success, and life-long achievement of students. The educational requirements for school nurses vary from state to state; however, the NASN recommends a baccalaureate degree in nursing from an accredited college or university and licensure as a registered nurse as the minimal preparation for the skills needed for entering school nursing practice (NASN, 2002). School nurses work with the students, parents or guardians, healthcare practitioners, teachers,

24 *Pediatric Nursing: Scope and Standards of Practice*

school administrators, and other professionals in the school setting and the community to provide or secure health services for children.

School nurses need to have expertise in clinical nursing, communication, surveillance, education, advocacy, and leadership in order to ensure that all students' health needs are addressed. The school nurse's role includes assessing the health status of students, identifying health problems that have an impact on health and learning, delivering emergency care, administering medications, performing healthcare procedures, providing wellness programs, advocating for children and families, and providing health counseling and health education. School nurses may be deemed first responders related to infectious disease outbreaks and episodes of violence or bioterrorism within and around the school. Overall, school nursing involves planning, developing, managing, and evaluating healthcare services to children in an educational setting and encompasses working with the families of the students and the community in which the student resides (Guilday, 2000; NASN & ANA, 2005).

School-based health centers (SBHCs) provide comprehensive physical and mental health services to children, with parental involvement, at locations accessible to children. SBHCs are not designed to replace an ongoing relationship a child may have with a primary provider, nor to replace the services of a school nurse. Rather, the SBHCs are designed to overcome existing social and economic barriers that prevent access to quality health care. Ideally, students receive comprehensive primary care, delivered in the context of family and community, which includes social services, mental health, and health education with a focus on wellness so that they may derive maximum benefit from their education (NAPNAP, 2005b). SBHCs should meet standards of care similar to those of community health centers, including certification and credentialing processes and a systematic evaluation of outcomes of services (Gance-Cleveland, Costin, & Degenstein, 2003).

These clinics are usually staffed by a pediatric nurse practitioner or physician's assistant, and a clinic assistant or receptionist, with access to a team of health educators, physicians, nutritionists, nurses, and social workers. The staff is trained to deal with the unique growth, social, developmental, and emotional needs of the school age population they serve. Activities of the school nurse or clinic may also include sponsoring health fairs and immunization programs, ongoing participation in crisis intervention teams, class health education, parent education,

Pediatric Nursing: Scope of Practice   **25**

teacher training, sports medicine clinics, student health clubs, question-and-answer columns in student newspapers, involvement in dropout prevention initiatives, and assessing health risk behaviors of the student population.

Pediatric nurses also provide health consultation to early care and education (ECE) programs (Crowley, 2001). The role of the child care health consultant (CCHC) is to minimize health risks and promote healthy behaviors in out-of-home care programs, and to link families with community-based health and developmental services (Ramler et al, 2006). Specifically, CCHCs promote health practices in ECE programs that may focus on nutrition, safe food handling, infection control, infant sleep position, monitoring of immunizations, and safe and active play. Evidence is emerging that the role of the CCHC can improve overall child care quality and school readiness among children (Ramler et al., 2006).

Transport Settings

Another setting for pediatric nursing practice is in air and surface transport. Neonates and infants who have increased acute care needs and technological support requirements may need air or surface transport from a community hospital or birth hospital to a facility with tertiary intensive capabilities. Young children and adolescents may require transport to a pediatric intensive care or other subspecialty unit. Pediatric specialty teams are typically composed of two RNs, an RN and NP, an RN and MD, or an RN with an MD and a Respiratory Therapist. The Air and Surface Transport Nurses Association (ASTNA) is a professional association for nurses working in the transport settings.

Camp Settings

Camp nursing affords the pediatric nurse the opportunity to provide all aspects of health care in an outdoor setting to either the general pediatric population or a specialty population (such as children with cancer, cystic fibrosis, asthma, diabetes, or developmental disabilities). The primary goal of the specialty camps is to allow the children, who may have had extensive or unpleasant medical treatment and life experiences, to enjoy a real camping experience while also learning about their illness or disability. Experienced pediatric nurses with current Basic Life Sup-

26   *Pediatric Nursing: Scope and Standards of Practice*

port training and Basic First Aid Training may choose to practice in camp settings. The Association of Camp Nurses has published a *Standards and Scope of Camp Nursing Practice* document (ACN, 2002) available for ordering at http://www.campnurse.org/store/acn.html.

Caring for a Diverse Population

Providing culturally competent care that values diversity, is based on self-assessment, and effectively manages the dynamics of differences between individuals and groups is fundamental to nursing practice. Due to the expanding cultural diversity of the American population, it is imperative that pediatric nurses understand and have a working knowledge of cultural characteristics and practices of the populations most served in their clinical area and are also aware of their own values and prejudices. Understanding cultural views can assist the pediatric nurse to anticipate and understand why and how families make certain decisions regarding their child's health. The pediatric nurse should expect that cultural and religious beliefs and practices may affect the management of the ill child, so these must be incorporated into the child and family care plan. When necessary, however, adjustments may need to be made when beliefs and practices are deemed unsafe for the child. For the pediatric nurse, it is imperative to apply knowledge of and demonstrate respect for culture and religion as a framework in the provision of care.

An appreciation of diversity and the promotion of inclusivity are also important when providing care to youth who are or think they may be gay, lesbian, bisexual, transgender, or who are struggling with or questioning their sexual orientation or gender identity (gay, lesbian, bisexual, transgender, and questioning; GLBTQ). Many GLBTQ youth are exposed to prejudice and encounter stigma, hostility or hatred which may hinder their ability to achieve developmental tasks (Harrison, 2003). These children tend to experience higher levels of isolation, runaway behavior, homelessness, domestic violence, depression, anxiety, suicide, violent victimization, substance abuse, and school or job failure as compared with heterosexual or gender-conforming youth (Nelson, 2003). Pediatric nurses should individualize interventions relating to health promotion and risk reduction for youth who identify or who are struggling whether to identify themselves as GLBTQ (NAPNAP, 2006a).

Pediatric Nursing: Scope of Practice   27

Global Perspectives of Pediatric Nursing

With the increasing ease at which people can travel worldwide, many opportunities exist for pediatric nursing globally. Many nurses travel to underdeveloped countries as part of their educational preparation in both undergraduate and graduate programs. Working in clinics, providing education and care to children and families, or serving as medical personnel for missionary teams are just some of the opportunities available to the pediatric generalist and advanced practice nurse. Through the International Council of Nursing (ICN), pediatric nurses can engage in or support larger global issues, such as quality nursing care for all, sound global health policies, the advancement of nursing knowledge, and the presence worldwide of a respected nursing profession and a competent and satisfied nursing workforce. While advances have been made in recent years in the fulfillment of children's rights to survival, health, and education, these gains are in danger of reversal in some parts of the world (Plotnick, 2007). On a global level, the predominant current risks to children are those stemming from poverty, environmental hazards, armed conflict, infectious diseases, and gender inequality.

Complementary Therapies

Increasingly, Americans are turning toward the use of complementary and alternative medicine (CAM) for themselves and their children. CAM is defined as a group of diverse medical and healthcare systems, practices, and products that are not presently considered as part of conventional medicine (National Center for Complementary and Alternative Medicine [NCCAM], 2007). This integrative approach combines conventional treatments with those for which there is high-quality evidence of safety and effectiveness. Examples of complementary and alternative therapies include mind–body techniques (meditation; prayer; creative expression through art, music, or dance), dietary supplements, herbal products, and manipulative or body-based practices such as massage, therapeutic touch, healing touch, Reiki, and magnetic field therapy (NCCAM, 2007). During the 1990s, the utilization of CAM increased from 11% in the early 1990s to 20% by the end of the decade (Ottolini et al., 1999). The use of these therapies for children with chronic illness or fatal conditions or diagnoses is estimated to range from 30–70% depending on patient age and access to service (Breuner, Barry, & Kemper 1998).

CAM is often used in conjunction with other diagnostic, treatment, or prevention strategies. Families who have had a negative experience with conventional medicine may choose alternative or complementary therapies, particularly for children with chronic illnesses. It is important for the pediatric healthcare provider to know what therapies patients and families are using, have a basic working knowledge of such treatments and providers, and be able to talk with families regarding the use of CAM therapies for their children. Also, it is important to assess whether the family has employed cultural practices, ethnic routines, or religious rituals that might include the use of herbs, medicines, or the wearing of certain charms.

Education

Education guidelines for the generalist level of pediatric nursing have been outlined in the *Standards and Guidelines for Pre-licensure and Professional Education for the Nursing Care of Children and Their Families* (Woodring & Pridham, 1998). This document was published with the intent of providing a new vision of education to prepare pre-licensure students and new graduates for the complex care of children and their families. The standards contain 11 concepts in three domains of knowledge and skills that are to be included in every educational program preparing nurses. The document does not produce the curriculum that should be provided within one specific course or set of courses about child health care. Rather, the standards state the goals, process criteria, and outcome criteria for the 11 concepts that can be integrated into all content areas and clinical settings where the needs of children and their families should be discussed. As a collaborator in developing this document, SPN strongly believes that the document serves as a guiding force to direct nursing education for the care of children in our complex society. Pediatric nurses, in collaboration with nursing faculty, help to provide key learning and clinical experiences for students.

Pre-licensure education for the generalist nurse may occur in a variety of programs including baccalaureate and graduate entry programs, associate degree programs, or perhaps a hospital diploma program. In 1986, the AACN published *The Essentials of Baccalaureate Education for Professional Nursing Practice,* a landmark set of core educational standards for the professional nurse. This document was updated in 1998 and is currently undergoing another revision to provide direction for the

Pediatric Nursing: Scope of Practice 29

education of professional nurses in the twenty-first century. *Essentials* defines the professional nurse as "that individual prepared with a minimum of a baccalaureate in nursing but is also inclusive of one who *enters* professional practice with a master's degree in nursing or a nursing doctorate" (AACN, 1998, p. 2).

Educational content regarding genomics and genetics has also been incorporated into nursing curricula. *Essential Nursing Competencies and Curricula Guidelines for Genetics and Genomics*, written by the Consensus Panel on Genetic/Genomic Competencies (2006), outlines the role of the nurse in applying and integrating genetic and genomic knowledge in the processes of screening, assessment, referral, and provision of education, care, and support. This document has been endorsed by numerous nursing organizations including the AAN, ANA, the National League for Nursing, NAPNAP, the National Association of Neonatal Nurses, the National Organization of Nurse Practitioner Faculty (NONPF) and SPN.

Post-baccalaureate education for the advanced practice pediatric nurse is required at the master's or doctoral level. In 1996, the AACN published *The Essentials of Master's Education for Advanced Practice Nursing*. This document outlines a generic core curriculum content for all advanced practice nursing students which includes research, policy, organization and financing of health care, ethics, professional role development, theoretical foundations of nursing practice, human diversity and social issues, and health promotion and disease prevention. A specialty core curriculum for APRNs who provide direct clinical care includes advanced health and physical assessment, advanced pathophysiology, and advanced pharmacology, in additional to clinical experiences.

The National Association of Clinical Nurse Specialists (NACNS) developed a *Statement on CNS Practice and Education* that provides a framework for a first level assessment of core CNS competencies regardless of specialty (NACNS, 2004). Similarly, NONPF (2006b) has developed curriculum guidelines for nurse practitioners, incorporating the full scope of advanced practice nursing. These guidelines and standards apply to graduate education and emphasize direct care across settings. The education of the advanced practice pediatric nurse includes specialty content in advanced health and physical assessment of the child, advanced physiology and pathophysiology, pediatric pharmacology, advanced

30   *Pediatric Nursing: Scope and Standards of Practice*

child and family development, family theory, promotion and maintenance of optimal health for children and families, and management of acute and chronic conditions in children.

Clinical practicum experiences for both CNSs and PNPs in a variety of settings are a vital part of the advanced practice curriculum. Clinical experience builds on course work and is designed to enable graduates to collect health data, establish a diagnosis, identify expected outcomes individualized to the child and family, plan and prescribe care, implement interventions, and evaluate the child's and family's progress toward attainment of outcomes. In clinical settings, students are expected to provide high-level nursing care based on current clinical evidence and guidelines and which incorporates technical skill, critical thinking, leadership, theoretical knowledge, and clinical scholarship. Academic faculty responsible for the overall implementation of advanced practice programs are ideally prepared at the doctoral level and are actively engaged in practice settings with children and families as clinicians, educators, or researchers. Preceptors actively collaborate with educators and students to guide clinical education. Preceptors are nurses who have demonstrated outstanding clinical expertise in a field related to pediatric advanced practice. In some academic institutions, preceptors may qualify for courtesy or clinical faculty appointments.

In the past decade, nurse leaders and educators examined the educational programs that prepare advanced practice nurses and reviewed reports and projections for the future healthcare needs of the twenty-first century. It was evident that the educational preparation and provision of services by advanced practice nurses coupled with the complexity of healthcare in the United States demanded a transformation. The recommendation was made by the AACN that the future education of advanced practice nurses (clinical nurse specialist and nurse practitioner) would occur at the doctoral level as a Doctor of Nursing Practice (DNP). ANCC recommends that this shift to doctoral preparation should occur by 2015. Additionally, many nurses have and will continue to obtain doctorate degrees in nursing science and education. These nurses are prepared for a wide range of practice environments and responsibilities, including advanced roles in academia, education, and research.

In preparing for this transition in education, the AACN charged a committee to develop *The Essentials of Doctoral Education for Advanced Nursing Practice* (AACN, 2006). This document incorporates and

Pediatric Nursing: Scope of Practice 31

Appendix B. Pediatric Nursing: Scope and Standards of Practice (2008)

expands on the *Master's Essentials*, currently used to guide advance practice education, to ensure the necessary academic and clinical rigor required for doctoral level education. The eight essentials for doctoral education include:

    I. Scientific underpinnings for practice

    II. Organizational and systems leadership for quality improvement and systems thinking

    III. Clinical scholarship and analytical methods for evidence-based practice

    IV. Information systems and technology, and patient care technology, for the improvement and transformation of health care

    V. Healthcare policy for advocacy in health care

    VI. Interprofessional collaboration for improving patient and population health outcomes

    VII. Clinical prevention and population health for improving the nation's health

    VIII. Advanced nursing practice

Additional work has been done to guide faculty in developing curricula and to set accreditation standards for programs. Advance practice nursing education will now align with audiology, medicine, pharmacy, and physical therapy in preparing practitioners with a terminal doctoral-level practice degree.

Certification

Certification is a process by which an independent, non-governmental agency recognizes an individual nurse's qualifications and knowledge for specialty nursing practice. All pediatric nurses should obtain certification. The nurse achieves specialty certification credentials through the completion of specialized education, experience in specialty nursing practice, and the successful completion of a qualifying examination. Continued certification is accomplished through a variety of mechanisms including re-examination, continuing education, self-assessment, and ongoing clinical practice. Through this process, the agency or professional organization acknowledges for the individual and to the

T A B L E 3 Pediatric Nursing Certification Opportunities

Certifying Organization	Certification Available
American Nurses Credentialing Center (ANCC)	Child/Adolescent Psychiatric and Mental Health Clinical Nurse Specialist, Pediatric Clinical Nurse Specialist, Pediatric Nurse, Pediatric Nurse Practitioner, School Nurse Practitioner*
American Association of Critical Care Nurses: AACCN Certification Corporation	Critical Care Registered Nurse – Pediatric (CCRN-P) Critical Care Registered Nurse – Neonatal (CCRN-N)
Corporation of Pediatric Oncology Nurses (CPON)	Certified Pediatric Oncology Nurse (CPON)
National Board for Certification of School Nurses (NBCSN)	National Certified School Nurse (NCSN)
National Certification Corporation (NCC)	Low-Risk Neonatal Nurse (RNC) Neonatal Intensive Care Nurse (RNC) Neonatal Nurse Practitioner (NNP)
Pediatric Nursing Certification Board (PNCB)	Certified Pediatric Nurse Practitioner – Primary Care (CPNP-PC) Certified Pediatric Nurse Practitioner – Acute Care (CPNP-AC) Certified Pediatric Nurse (CPN)

* Certification is no longer offered

general public that the nurse has mastered a body of knowledge for a particular specialty. Certification is evolving with multiple opportunities for certification available (see Table 3). The nurse should be informed about which certification option is appropriate for him or her.

Regulation

Professional certification is required to practice as a nurse practitioner in most states (Pearson, 2007). State jurisdictions have regulatory and legal oversight of practice for the RN and APRN. There is considerable variability among states in the implementation of this oversight, and APRN statutes vary widely from title protection to a more specific delineation of APRN practice. The autonomy of practice ranges from

Pediatric Nursing: Scope of Practice 33

private practice with referral options to practicing under the supervision of a physician. The ANA supports one scope of nursing practice, one licensure for registered nurses, and minimal statutory language about advanced practice. The ANA also proposes that state constituent member associations promote specific designations of APRN roles in rules and regulations instead of law to avoid attaching statutory language to the roles. Additionally, the profession should develop consistent standards of regulation through certification, peer review, and continuing education to self-regulate the role so that the profession retains the responsibility and accountability for regulating practice.

Professional Issues and Trends

Within the broad context of rising healthcare costs, the increasing number of uninsured children and families in the United States, and the consequent disparities in the delivery of health care to those in need, the current professional issues and trends for pediatric nurses are as varied as the settings in which they practice. In acute care and inpatient settings, children with complex diseases are surviving longer, thereby creating new adolescent and young adult populations still needing follow-up care by pediatric healthcare providers in pediatric inpatient units. Thus, creating the need for ongoing education in the areas of adult medicine. Also, many pediatric providers work with chronically ill adolescents in a variety of settings during their transition to adulthood.

With the development of new vaccines, the percentage of pediatric inpatient admissions for infectious disease has declined. As noted above, more parents are turning towards the use of CAM therapies as an adjunct to conventional medical treatments in treating their children. For advanced practice pediatric nurses in primary and specialty care settings, additional clinical challenges include providing care for children who present with chronic health problems that stem from complications of overweight and obesity, asthma and allergic conditions, and behavioral and mental health concerns.

More children's hospitals are seeking Magnet Status from the American Nurses Credentialing Center (ANCC), which identifies institutions as meeting set standards for the provision of excellent nursing care. Because of this pursuit, pediatric nurses in both general and advanced practice are seeking certification and advanced educational degrees.

34   *Pediatric Nursing: Scope and Standards of Practice*

Professionally, nurses continue to address issues of entry into practice, the autonomy of advanced practice, multiple certification pathways, and the various educational credentials appropriate for certification. Overall, efforts must be made to narrow the gap between the abilities of healthcare providers and the activities which governmental regulation prevents them from performing (Safriet 2002). Nurses must continue to demonstrate to the payers of health care and to the public the value of an interdisciplinary system which provides efficient, quality health care.

Ethical Issues in Pediatric Care

Pediatric care is delivered in an environment of specialized knowledge and skill under circumstances in which opportunities for ethical deliberation and reflection may be less than ideal. Parents and families are emotionally stressed, and in some instances they themselves may be patients. Staffing and other organizational issues may introduce additional stress on the care team apart from the dynamics of a particular case. These examples only emphasize the importance of viewing the pediatric care unit as a moral community in which ethical reflection, discussion, and action are as much a part of a care plan as diagnosis and treatment. Viewing ethics in this context also allows for an understanding of ethical issues that is both deep and broad, encompassing ethical distress that may occur within one's self, among members of the care team, and between the care team and families.

The values of advocacy, respect for persons, and justice are among those that have been identified by nurses as societal values with particular relevance to the profession of nursing. Thus, as a member of the profession, each individual nurse has accepted the ethical obligations of the role in addition to the individual capacity to make moral choices as human beings. While this provides a rich legacy, it can also be a source of ethical uncertainty or conflict when the care plan for a particular patient or institutional rules require some sacrifice of one's individual moral code in carrying out professional responsibilities. In some cases, a healthy professional distance allows us to carry out decisions that are ethically permissible even though they are not the choices we would make for our own children.

Occasionally, however, a case presents itself in which taking this course is not easily reconciled. Prolonged life-supporting therapy that

Pediatric Nursing: Scope of Practice   35

Appendix B. Pediatric Nursing: Scope and Standards of Practice (2008)

is insisted on by parents and allowed by physicians may in some cases compromise both a nurse's professional identity and personal moral agency. How such situations are handled is as ethically important as the course of action one chooses to take.

How pediatric nurses understand what an ethical dilemma is can influence their ability to identify ethical issues, discuss them with colleagues, and take action to resolve or ameliorate ethical conflict. Differences within the healthcare team may be enriched or impeded by different cultural and religious backgrounds and by hierarchical and power differentials that are often unspoken but powerful influences in how a unit functions. Understanding the unit as a moral community includes not only how we treat patients, but also how nurses treat each other. All members of the healthcare team must have a realistic under-standing of ethics as an everyday concern rather than an issue of crisis management, so that an environment is created in which high standards are the rule rather than the exception, providing support for a commu-nity characterized by mutual respect and willingness to take responsi-bility for lapses and improvements.

Although there is a tendency to put difficult cases behind oneself as quickly as possible and move on, ethical growth requires that nurses reflect on our practice so that one can identify and reinforce what one does well and learn from one's inexperience and mistakes. Nursing codes of ethics provide principles based on important moral values that shape the nurse's professional identity (ANA, 2001) and provide the nurse the foundation to apply the principles in his or her work setting.

Advocacy in Pediatric Care

Every pediatric nurse is a child advocate. Advocacy can occur in the hospital setting, ambulatory care setting, educational setting, commit-tee meetings, agency discussions, parent meetings, and public settings, sometimes on a daily basis. Advocacy means providing a voice for those who are not heard, ensuring that important issues are addressed (Sullivan 2004). Pediatric nurses hold many qualities that are needed for advocating: strong communication skills, the ability to negotiate, awareness of patient needs, perseverance, leadership and people skills, and the ability to both multitask and think innovatively "outside the workplace". The specialized knowledge that pediatric nurses possess, combined with their holistic approach and their understanding of the context of child health, can assist in the creation, implementation, and evaluation of policies at all levels. Pediatric nurses can be involved in advocacy by finding their passion related to their work, community, or personal interests which can all lead to avenues of advocacy. Being involved in committees in the workplace, committees for professional associations, and involvement in community activities are examples of advocacy opportunities.

Pediatric nurses understand both the pediatric patient and family needs, which places them in a prime position to advocate for those identified needs. Because of their expertise, the pediatric nurse can see the effects of policy decisions on the health and well-being of the patient and family. Professional values of possessing an ethical framework, abiding by the code of ethics for nurses (ANA, 2001), and acknowledging the mission and goals of professional organizations can guide the nurse in advocacy efforts. Advocacy success has been demonstrated in areas surrounding the development of safe playgrounds, choking prevention, ensuring healthier school lunch programs, and assuring funding and services in state children's health insurance programs (SCHIP).

Continued Commitment to the Profession

Pediatric healthcare professionals are committed to:

- demonstrating excellent nursing practice consistent with professional nursing standards, specialty nursing standards, and state boards of registered nursing regulations for generalist and advanced practice nurses;
- supporting education and role development of novice practitioners by serving as preceptors, role models, and mentors;
- advancing the profession through enhancing public awareness and community activities;
- maintaining active membership in professional organizations;
- working to influence policy-making bodies to improve access to quality health care;
- using an ethical framework to evaluate issues regarding care; and

Pediatric Nursing: Scope of Practice 37

Appendix B. Pediatric Nursing: Scope and Standards of Practice (2008)

- demonstrating practice consistent with ethical and legal standards in compliance with state and federal regulations.

Furthermore, pediatric nurses are committed to working together to address the common issues that affect pediatric nurses who practice in diverse roles and settings and who may belong to varied professional pediatric organizations. In so doing, they are able to effectively merge their knowledge, insights, resources, and goals for the future, and thereby improve the health care of the children and families to whom they are ultimately accountable.

38   *Pediatric Nursing: Scope and Standards of Practice*

STANDARDS OF PEDIATRIC NURSING PRACTICE
STANDARDS OF PRACTICE

STANDARD 1. ASSESSMENT
The pediatric nurse collects comprehensive data pertinent to the patient's health or the situation.

Measurement Criteria:

The Pediatric Nurse:

- Collects data in a systematic and ongoing process that conveys respect for the child and family.

- Involves the child, family, other individuals important to the family, and other healthcare providers, as appropriate, in holistic data collection.

- Utilizes the preferred language of the family through a culturally sensitive process, and seeks a qualified interpreter if necessary.

- Assesses the child's and family's environment.

- Prioritizes data collection activities based on the child's immediate condition, situation, and anticipated needs.

- Uses appropriate evidence-based assessment techniques specific for the child's age in collecting pertinent data.

  - Physical assessment may include but not be limited to:

    - Height, weight (current and pre-illness), body mass index (BMI)

    - Vital signs including pain assessment

    - Hearing and vision screening

    - Tanner staging of pubertal development

    - Nutritional status

    - Physical examination

    - Head circumference (age-appropriate)

Continued ▶

39

Appendix B. Pediatric Nursing: Scope and Standards of Practice (2008)

- Behavioral assessment may include but not be limited to:
  - Tolerance of the physical examination or procedures
  - Affect and activity
  - Interactions with adults and peers
  - Behavioral differences across settings (home, school, clinic, hospital)
- Developmental assessment may include but not be limited to:
  - Personal characteristics and social skills
  - Language
  - Fine motor and adaptive
  - Gross motor
  - Cognitive
  - Emotional and mental health
  - Temperament
  - Moral development
- Family assessment may include:
  - Determining who the child lives with
  - Familial strengths
  - Cultural background
  - Ethnic background
  - Socioeconomic background
  - Mental health issues
  - Religious or spiritual background
  - Coping strategies
  - Learning style
  - Injury prevention and safety practices
  - Preferences of family for receiving information and support
  - Ways the family can partner in providing the child's health care

Appendix B. Pediatric Nursing: Scope and Standards of Practice (2008)

The content in this appendix is not current and is of historical significance only.

- Health history may include but not be limited to:
  - Birth history (age-appropriate)
  - Growth and development milestones
  - Past medical illness or surgeries
  - Medications and allergies
  - Family history, including genetic history and congenital abnormalities
  - Mental or emotional disabilities, metabolic problems, and chronic health problems
  - Accidents or injuries
  - Educational needs related to maximizing the child's health
  - Behavioral patterns and individual strengths
  - Communicable or childhood diseases
  - Exposure to hazardous agents
  - Dietary habits and intake history
  - Growth parameters as compared with normal for age
  - Significant trends in weight gain or loss
  - Immunization status
  - Sexual history (age-appropriate)
  - Substance abuse history (age-appropriate)
  - Engagement in high-risk activities (smoking, drugs or alcohol, body piercing or tattoos, sexual activity, performance-enhancing drugs)
  - Experience with pain and pain management techniques
  - School history (age-appropriate)
  - Elimination patterns
  - Sleep patterns and sleep aids
  - Information that family member sees as significant

Continued ▶

Standards of Pediatric Nursing Practice 41

Appendix B. Pediatric Nursing: Scope and Standards of Practice (2008)

- Family observations of the child
- Strengths of the child and family
- Any significant stressors; comforting and coping strategies
- Relationships with the family, including potential for abuse
- Socioeconomic, cultural, spiritual, and environmental factors
- Peer relationships
- Travel history

- Uses analytical models and problem-solving tools to systematically collect data.
- Synthesizes available data, information, and knowledge relevant to the situation to identify patterns and variances.
- Documents relevant data in a retrievable form.
- Bases assessment techniques on research and knowledge, using clinical judgment to ensure that relevant and necessary data are collected.

Additional Measurement Criteria for the Advanced Practice Pediatric Nurse:

The Advanced Practice Pediatric Nurse:

- Initiates and interprets age-appropriate and condition-specific laboratory tests and diagnostic procedures.

42   *Pediatric Nursing: Scope and Standards of Practice*

STANDARD 2. DIAGNOSIS

The pediatric nurse analyzes the assessment data to determine the diagnoses or healthcare issues.

Measurement Criteria:

The Pediatric Nurse:

- Derives the diagnoses or issues based on assessment data.

- Derives diagnoses that are developmentally appropriate and specific to areas of growth and development, age, cultural sensitivity, and family dynamics.

- Validates the prioritized diagnoses or issues with the child, family, significant others, and other healthcare providers when possible and appropriate.

- Documents diagnoses or issues in a manner that facilitates the determination of the expected outcomes and plan of care.

Additional Measurement Criteria for the Advanced Practice Pediatric Nurse:

The Advanced Practice Pediatric Nurse:

- Systematically compares and contrasts clinical findings with normal and abnormal variations and developmental events in formulating a differential diagnosis.

- Determines diagnoses related to disease and injury prevention and health promotion, restoration, and maintenance.

- Utilizes complex data and information obtained during interview, examination, and diagnostic procedures in identifying diagnoses.

- Revises diagnoses as appropriate to the ongoing evaluation.

- Conforms diagnosis to an accepted classification system (as may be defined by the healthcare setting).

- Assists staff in developing and maintaining competency in the diagnostic process.

Standards of Pediatric Nursing Practice 43

STANDARD 3. OUTCOMES IDENTIFICATION
The pediatric nurse identifies expected outcomes for a plan of care individualized to the child, family, and the situation.

Measurement Criteria:

The Pediatric Nurse:

- Involves the child (when age appropriate), family, and other healthcare providers in formulating expected outcomes when possible and appropriate.

- Derives outcomes that are developmentally appropriate, age-specific, family centered, and culturally sensitive.

- Derives outcomes that are realistic in relation to the child's and family's potential capabilities and available resources.

- Considers associated risks, benefits, costs, current scientific evidence, and clinical expertise when formulating expected outcomes.

- Defines expected outcomes in terms of the child, the child's values, ethical considerations, environment or situation with consideration of risks, benefits and costs, and current scientific evidence.

- Includes a time estimate for attainment of expected outcomes, and prioritizes as appropriate.

- Develops expected outcomes that provide direction for continuity of care.

- Identifies expected outcomes that incorporate scientific evidence and are achievable through implementation of evidence-based practices.

- Modifies expected outcomes based on changes in the status of the child or evaluation of the situation.

- Documents expected outcomes as measurable goals.

Additional Measurement Criteria for the Advanced Practice Pediatric Nurse:

The Advanced Practice Pediatric Nurse:

- Identifies expected outcomes with consideration of the associated risks, benefits, and costs for the child and family.

44   _**Pediatric Nursing: Scope and Standards of Practice**_

- Identifies expected outcomes that incorporate cost and clinical effectiveness, the child's and family's satisfaction, and continuity and consistency among providers.

- Supports the use of clinical guidelines linked to positive outcomes for the child.

Standards of Pediatric Nursing Practice   45

STANDARD 4. PLANNING

The pediatric nurse develops a plan of care that prescribes strategies and alternatives to attain expected outcomes.

Measurement Criteria:

The Pediatric Nurse:

- Develops an individualized plan of care considering the child's characteristics or the situation (including age, growth, developmental, cultural, and environmental factors).

- Develops the plan of care in conjunction with the child (when developmentally able), family, and others, as appropriate.

- Formulates a plan of care that is family centered and reflects current pediatric nursing practice, and takes into consideration the family's cultural needs, ability to read and write, level of health literacy, and capacity for understanding complex healthcare processes.

- Includes strategies within the plan of care that address each of the identified diagnoses or issues, which may include strategies for promotion and restoration of health and prevention of illness, injury, and disease.

- Provides for continuity within the plan of care.

- Provides for confidentiality when necessary.

- Incorporates an implementation pathway or timeline within the plan of care that is dynamic, flexible, and reassessed as needed.

- Re-evaluates the plan of care with the child, family, and others as appropriate.

- Utilizes the plan of care to provide direction to other members of the healthcare team.

- Defines the plan of care to reflect current statutes, rules and regulations, and standards.

- Integrates current trends and research affecting care in the planning process.

- Considers the economic impact of the plan of care.

The content in this appendix is not current and is of historical significance only.

- Uses standardized language or recognized terminology to document the plan of care.
- Documents the plan of care.

Additional Measurement Criteria for the Advanced Practice Pediatric Nurse:

The Advanced Practice Pediatric Nurse:

- Identifies assessment, diagnostic strategies, and therapeutic interventions within the plan of care that reflect current pediatric healthcare practice, including data, research, literature, and expert clinical knowledge.

- Devises a comprehensive plan of care that reflects the responsibilities of the advanced practice nurse, the child, and the family and may include delegation of responsibilities and consultation to assist others in implementing the plan of care.

- Participates in the design and development of multidisciplinary and interdisciplinary processes to address the situation or issue.

- Formulates the comprehensive plan of care that includes educational interventions related to the child's health status, conventional and alternative therapies, self-care activities, and appropriate referrals and coordination of comprehensive services to ensure continuity of care.

- Documents the comprehensive plan of care in a manner that allows access by the child, the family, and healthcare providers as appropriate, and provides direction for the family and the healthcare team as they focus on attaining expected outcomes.

- Selects or designs strategies to meet the multifaceted needs of the complex pediatric patient.

- Includes the synthesis of the child's and family's values and beliefs regarding nursing and medical therapies within the plan of care.

- Contributes to the development and continuous improvement of organizational systems that support the plan of care process.

- Supports the integration of clinical, human, and financial resources to enhance and complete the decision-making processes.

Standards of Pediatric Nursing Practice 47

Appendix B. Pediatric Nursing: Scope and Standards of Practice (2008)

Standard 5. Implementation
The pediatric nurse implements the identified plan of care.

Measurement Criteria:

The Pediatric Nurse:

- Performs interventions that are consistent with the established plan of care and are family centered, developmentally appropriate, age specific, and culturally sensitive.

- Encourages the child of accountable age and ability to assume responsibility related to his or her care.

- Provides to the child or the caregiver education that includes health promotion, anticipatory guidance, information about injury and disease prevention, and home care management as appropriate for the child's developmental level.

- Counsels the child and family in resolving issues or making determinations of what the next appropriate steps might be. Implements the plan of care in a safe, cost-effective, and timely manner.

- Documents implementation and any modifications, including changes or omissions, of the identified plan of care.

- Utilizes evidence-based interventions and treatments specific to the diagnosis or problem.

- Utilizes community resources and systems to implement the plan of care, and coordinates access to the appropriate resources.

- Collaborates with nursing colleagues and others to implement the plan of care.

Additional Measurement Criteria for the Advanced Practice Pediatric Nurse:

The Advanced Practice Pediatric Nurse:

- Facilitates utilization of systems and community resources to implement the plan of care.

- Supports collaboration with nursing colleagues and other disciplines to implement the plan of care.

- Incorporates new knowledge and strategies to initiate change in nursing care practices if desired outcomes are not achieved.

The content in this appendix is not current and is of historical significance only.

- Implements interventions and treatments that are based on current clinical evidence and theory.

- Performs interventions and treatments for which the nurse has received appropriate training and has demonstrated competency in the skill or procedure being performed.

- Implements the plan of care using principles and concepts of project or systems management.

- Fosters organizational systems that support implementation of the plan of care.

Standards of Pediatric Nursing Practice   49

Standard 5a: Coordination of Care and Case Management
The pediatric nurse coordinates care delivery.

Measurement Criteria:

The Pediatric Nurse:

- Coordinates implementation of the plan of care.
- Documents the coordination of the care.
- Communicates with all healthcare providers involved in the child's care.

Additional Measurement Criteria for the Advanced Practice Pediatric Nurse:

The Advanced Practice Pediatric Nurse:

- Provides leadership in the coordination of multidisciplinary health care for integrated delivery of pediatric care services.
- Delegates appropriate monitoring, assessments, and interventions according to the condition of the child and the relative skill and scope of practice of the caregiver.
- Provides case management and clinical coordination of care using sophisticated data synthesis with consideration of the child's and family's complex needs and desired outcomes.
- Coordinates system and community resources to achieve optimal quality of care, delivered in a cost-effective manner within an inter-disciplinary team approach.
- Negotiates health-related services and additional specialized care with the child, the family, appropriate systems, agencies, and providers across continuums of care.

STANDARD 5B: HEALTH TEACHING AND HEALTH PROMOTION, RESTORATION AND MAINTENANCE

The pediatric nurse employs strategies to promote health and a safe environment.

Measurement Criteria:

The Pediatric Nurse:

- Provides health teaching that addresses such topics as healthy lifestyles, risk-reducing behaviors, developmental needs, activities of daily living, and preventive self-care and is based on current scientific knowledge, research, epidemiological principles, and the family's health beliefs and practices.

- Uses health promotion and health teaching methods appropriate to the situation and to the child's and family's developmental levels, learning needs, readiness, ability to learn, language preference, and culture.

- Provides information on the risks and benefits of healthcare practices.

- Seeks opportunities for feedback and evaluation of the effectiveness of the strategies used.

- Designs health information and pediatric education appropriate to the child's culture, age, developmental and cognitive levels, and readiness and ability to learn.

- Evaluates health information resources, such as the Internet, within the area of practice for accuracy, readability, and comprehensibility to help the child and the family access quality health information.

Additional Measurement Criteria for the Advanced Practice Pediatric Nurse:

The Advanced Practice Pediatric Nurse:

- Employs diverse and complex strategies, interventions, and teaching with the child and the family to promote, maintain, restore, and improve health, and to prevent illness and injury.

Continued ▶

Standards of Pediatric Nursing Practice 51

Appendix B. Pediatric Nursing: Scope and Standards of Practice (2008)

STANDARDS OF PRACTICE

- Synthesizes empirical evidence on risk behaviors, learning theories, behavioral change theories, motivational theories, epidemiology, and other related theories and frameworks when designing health information and pediatric education.

- Bases anticipatory guidance and teaching on current scientific knowledge, research, epidemiological principles, and the family's health beliefs and practices.

- Provides the child (if age appropriate) and the family information regarding the interventions including potential benefits, risks, complications, and alternatives.

Standard 5c: Consultation

The pediatric nurse provides consultation to healthcare providers and others to influence the identified plan of care for children, to enhance the abilities of others to provide health care, and to effect change in the healthcare system.

Measurement Criteria:

The Pediatric Nurse:

- Synthesizes data, information, theoretical frameworks, and evidence when providing consultation.

- Facilitates the effectiveness of a consultation by involving the stakeholders in the decision-making process.

- Communicates consultation recommendations that influence the identified plan of care, facilitate understanding by involved stakeholders, enhance the work of others, and effect change.

Additional Measurement Criteria for the Advanced Practice Pediatric Nurse:

The Advanced Practice Pediatric Nurse:

- Bases consultative activities on theoretical frameworks, including those that focus on family systems and family-centered care, and on evidence for best practice.

- Bases consultation on mutual respect among the child, the family, and other primary caregivers.

- Initiates consultation through mutual identification of the needs for intervention and problem identification

- Initiates appropriate consultation to implement the interdisciplinary plan of care for the child with consideration given to the child's unique developmental needs and abilities and the family's level of adaptation and ability to cope with the child's health concerns.

- Communicates consultation recommendations in terms that facilitate change.

- Supports the child and the family in their decision-making regarding the implementation of the plan of care.

Standards of Pediatric Nursing Practice   53

STANDARDS OF PRACTICE

STANDARD 5D: PRESCRIPTIVE AUTHORITY AND TREATMENT

The Advanced Practice Pediatric Nurse utilizes prescriptive authority, procedures, referrals, treatments, and therapies in providing care.

Measurement Criteria for the Advanced Practice Pediatric Nurse:

The Advanced Practice Pediatric Nurse:

- Prescribes evidence-based treatments, therapies, and procedures considering the child's comprehensive healthcare needs and based on current pediatric knowledge, research, and practice.

- Prescribes appropriate non-pharmacological interventions, including complementary and alternative therapies.

- Performs procedures as needed in the delivery of comprehensive care to the child.

- Prescribes pharmacologic agents based on current knowledge of pharmacological and physiological principles that are both universal and unique to the care of children at each stage in their development.

- Prescribes specific pharmacological agents and treatments based on clinical indicators, the child's status and needs, and the results of diagnostic and laboratory tests.

- Provides the child (if age appropriate) and family with information about diagnostic and laboratory results, as well as effects and potential adverse effects of proposed prescriptive therapies.

- Evaluates therapeutic and potential adverse effects of pharmacological and non-pharmacological treatments.

- Provides information to the family regarding agents the child should refrain from taking because of the potential adverse effects on the child.

- Provides the child (if age appropriate) and family with information about costs, alternative treatments, and procedures, as appropriate.

- Monitors current issues related to pharmacological agents, including off-label use and pediatric safe dosage for medications indicated for adults.

54   *Pediatric Nursing: Scope and Standards of Practice*

STANDARD 5E: REFERRAL

The Advanced Practice Pediatric Nurse identifies the need for additional care and makes referrals as indicated.

Measurement Criteria:

The Advanced Practice Pediatric Nurse:

- Discusses referrals with the child (if age appropriate) and family.

- Makes referrals to other healthcare providers and community service agencies as appropriate to the needs of the child with consideration of benefits and costs.

- Ensures continuity of care throughout the healthcare referral process by implementing recommendations from referral sources.

- Identifies and coordinates access to appropriate community resources.

Standards of Pediatric Nursing Practice

55

STANDARDS OF PRACTICE

STANDARD 6. EVALUATION

The pediatric nurse evaluates progress towards attainment of outcomes.

Measurement Criteria:

The Pediatric Nurse:

- Conducts a systematic, ongoing, and criterion-based evaluation of the outcomes in relation to the structures and processes prescribed by the plan of care and the indicated timeline.

- Includes the child, family, and other healthcare providers involved in the care or situation in the evaluation process.

- Evaluates the effectiveness of the plan of care strategies in relation to the child's responses and the attainment of the expected outcomes.

- Documents the results of the evaluation.

- Uses ongoing assessment data to revise the diagnoses, outcomes, the plan of care, and the implementation as needed.

- Documents revisions in diagnoses, outcomes, and the plan of care.

- Documents the child's and the family's readiness for and responses to interventions.

- Disseminates evaluation results to the child (if age appropriate), the family, and others involved in the care or situation, as appropriate.

Additional Measurement Criteria for the Advanced Practice Pediatric Nurse:

The Advanced Practice Pediatric Nurse:

- Evaluates the accuracy of the diagnosis and effectiveness of the interventions in relationship to the child's attainment of expected outcomes.

- Bases the evaluation process on advanced knowledge, practice, and research about child health care.

- Utilizes results of evaluation analyses to revise or resolve the diagnoses, expected outcomes, and plan of care.

56   *Pediatric Nursing: Scope and Standards of Practice*

- Synthesizes the results of the evaluation analyses to determine the impact of the plan of care on the affected child, family, groups, communities, institutions, networks, and organizations

- Utilizes the results of the evaluation analyses to make or recommend process or structural changes including policy, procedure, or protocol documentation as appropriate.

Appendix B. Pediatric Nursing: Scope and Standards of Practice (2008)

The content in this appendix is not current and is of historical significance only.

STANDARDS OF PROFESSIONAL PERFORMANCE

STANDARD 7. QUALITY OF PRACTICE
The pediatric nurse systematically enhances the quality and effectiveness of nursing practice.

Measurement Criteria:

The Pediatric Nurse:

- Demonstrates quality by documenting the application of the nursing process and evidence-based practice in a responsible, accountable, and ethical manner.

- Uses the results of quality improvement activities to initiate changes in pediatric nursing practice and in the healthcare delivery system, and communicates results to others who may benefit.

- Uses creativity and innovation in pediatric nursing practice to improve care delivery to children and families.

- Incorporates new knowledge to initiate changes in nursing practice if desired outcomes are not achieved.

- Participates in quality improvement activities. Such activities may include:

  - Identifying aspects of practice important for quality monitoring.

  - Using indicators developed to monitor quality and effectiveness of nursing practice.

  - Collecting data to monitor quality and effectiveness of nursing practice.

  - Analyzing quality data to identify opportunities for improving nursing practice.

  - Formulating recommendations to improve nursing practice or outcomes.

  - Developing, implementing, and evaluating activities, policies, procedures, and guidelines to improve the quality of practice.

Continued ▶

59

- Participating on interdisciplinary teams to improve the care delivery process and patient outcomes.
- Participating in efforts to minimize costs and unnecessary duplication.
- Analyzing factors related to safety, satisfaction, effectiveness, and cost–benefit options.
- Analyzing organizational systems for barriers.
- Implementing processes to remove or decrease barriers within organizational systems.

Additional Measurement Criteria for the Advanced Practice Pediatric Nurse:

The Advanced Practice Pediatric Nurse:

- Designs quality improvement initiatives.
- Implements initiatives to evaluate the need for change.
- Evaluates the practice environment and quality of nursing care rendered in relation to existing evidence, identifying opportunities for the generation and translation of research findings.
- Obtains and maintains professional certification in advanced practice pediatric nursing.
- Provides leadership in establishing and monitoring standards of practice to improve care of children and their families in collaboration with other healthcare team members.
- Participates in efforts to minimize costs and unnecessary duplication of tests and diagnostic services, and facilitates the timely provision of services for the child and the family.
- Analyzes factors related to safety, satisfaction, effectiveness, and cost–benefit options with the child, family, and other healthcare providers as appropriate.
- Identifies and works to remove barriers in organizational systems that may hinder the quality of pediatric nursing care.

Appendix B. Pediatric Nursing: Scope and Standards of Practice (2008)

Appendix B. *Pediatric Nursing: Scope and Standards of Practice (2008)*

STANDARD 8. PROFESSIONAL PRACTICE EVALUATION
The pediatric nurse evaluates one's own nursing practice in relation to professional practice standards and guidelines, relevant statutes, rules, and regulations.

Measurement Criteria:

The Pediatric Nurse:

- Evaluates one's own cultural and ethnic sensitivity when providing care.

- Engages in self-evaluation of practice on a regular basis, identifying areas of strength as well as areas in which professional development would be beneficial.

- Obtains informal feedback regarding one's own practice from the child and family, peers, professional colleagues, and others.

- Participates in systematic peer review as appropriate.

- Takes action to achieve goals identified during the evaluation process.

- Provides rationale for practice beliefs, decisions, and actions as part of the informal and formal evaluation processes.

- Applies knowledge of current professional practice standards, guidelines, statutes, rules, and regulations that affect the nursing care of children and families.

- Evaluates performance according to the standards of the profession and the standards specific to pediatric nursing and various regulatory bodies, and takes action to improve practice.

- Analyzes the effectiveness of interventions, the incidence and types of complications, and child outcome data to improve practice.

- Takes action to achieve goals identified during performance appraisal and peer review, resulting in changes in practice and role performance.

- Synthesizes and uses the results of evaluation to make or recommend changes including policy, procedure, or protocol documentation.

Continued ▶

Standards of Pediatric Nursing Practice 61

The content in this appendix is not current and is of historical significance only.

Additional Measurement Criteria for the Advanced Practice Pediatric Nurse:

The Advanced Practice Pediatric Nurse:

- Engages in a formal process seeking feedback regarding one's own practice from the child, family, peers, professional colleagues, and others.

STANDARD 9. EDUCATION
The pediatric nurse attains knowledge and competency that reflects current nursing practice.

Measurement Criteria:

The Pediatric Nurse:

- Participates in ongoing nursing and interdisciplinary educational activities related to clinical knowledge and professional issues.

- Demonstrates a commitment to lifelong learning through self-reflection and inquiry to identify learning needs.

- Seeks experiences that reflect current pediatric nursing practice in order to maintain skills and competence in clinical practice or role performance.

- Acquires culturally competent and clinically sound knowledge and skills appropriate to the health care of children and their families, and to the practice setting, role, or situation.

- Maintains professional records that provide evidence of competency and lifelong learning.

- Seeks experiences as well as formal and independent learning activities to maintain and develop clinical and professional skills and knowledge.

Additional Measurement Criteria for the Advanced Practice Pediatric Nurse:

The Advanced Practice Pediatric Nurse:

- Utilizes current healthcare research findings and other evidence to expand clinical knowledge, enhance role performance, and increase knowledge of professional issues.

- Supports the education and role development of other practitioners by serving as preceptor, role model, and mentor.

Standards of Pediatric Nursing Practice 63

Appendix B. Pediatric Nursing: Scope and Standards of Practice (2008)

STANDARD 10. COLLEGIALITY

The pediatric nurse interacts with and contributes to the professional development of peers and colleagues.

Measurement Criteria:

The Pediatric Nurse:

- Shares knowledge and skills with peers and colleagues as evidenced by such activities as child care conferences or presentations at formal or informal meetings.

- Provides peers with feedback regarding their practice and role performance.

- Interacts with peers and colleagues to enhance one's own professional nursing practice and role performance.

- Maintains compassionate and caring relationships with peers and colleagues.

- Contributes to an environment that is conducive to the clinical education of nursing students and other healthcare professionals.

- Contributes to a supportive and healthy work environment.

Additional Measurement Criteria for the Advanced Practice Pediatric Nurse:

The Advanced Practice Pediatric Nurse:

- Models expert practice to interdisciplinary team members and healthcare consumers.

- Participates on interdisciplinary teams that contribute to role development, advanced pediatric nursing practice, and health care.

- Contributes to an environment that is conducive to clinical education of other healthcare providers, including teaching, mentoring, and precepting.

- Contributes to the professional development of others to improve child health care and to foster the profession's growth.

STANDARD 11. COLLABORATION
The pediatric nurse collaborates with the child, family, and others in the conduct of nursing practice.

Measurement Criteria:

The Pediatric Nurse:

- Communicates with child, family, and others regarding health care of the child and the nurse's role in providing that care.

- Collaborates with the interdisciplinary and intradisciplinary health-care teams and family in creating a documented plan of care focusing on outcomes and decisions related to patient care and delivery of services.

- Partners with others to effect change and generate positive outcomes through knowledge of the child or situation.

- Documents referrals, including provision for continuity of care.

- Assists the family in identifying and accessing community resources to support the family in the care of the child as appropriate.

Additional Measurement Criteria for the Advanced Practice Pediatric Nurse:

The Advanced Practice Pediatric Nurse:

- Partners with other disciplines to enhance pediatric health care through interdisciplinary activities, such as education, consultation, development of new management and therapeutic strategies or research.

- Facilitates an interdisciplinary process with other members of the healthcare team.

- Documents plans, communications, management plan changes, and collaborative discussions to improve pediatric health care.

The content in this appendix is not current and is of historical significance only.

Standards of Pediatric Nursing Practice 65

STANDARD 12. ETHICS

The pediatric nurse integrates ethical considerations and processes in all areas of practice.

Measurement Criteria:

The Pediatric Nurse:

- Uses *Code of Ethics for Nurses with Interpretive Statements* (ANA 2001) to guide practice.
- Delivers care in a manner that preserves and protects the child's and family's autonomy, dignity, and rights.
- Delivers care in a nonjudgmental and nondiscriminatory manner that is sensitive to and values diversity.
- Maintains confidentiality within legal and regulatory parameters.
- Enables children and families to participate in ethical decision-making processes.
- Maintains a therapeutic and professional relationship with appropriate professional role boundaries.
- Demonstrates a commitment to practicing self-care, managing stress, and connecting with self and others.
- Facilitates family participation in ethical decision-making.
- Contributes to multidisciplinary teams or committees that address ethical questions, benefits, and outcomes.
- Informs administrators or others of the risks, benefits, and outcomes of programs and decisions that affect healthcare delivery.
- Reports abuse of patients' rights and incompetent, unethical, or illegal practice.

Additional Measurement Criteria for the Advanced Practice Pediatric Nurse:

The Advanced Practice Pediatric Nurse:

- Ensures that the care provided is consistent with the child's and family's needs and values, and with codes of ethical practice.
- Informs the child (as appropriate) and family of the risks, benefits, and outcomes of healthcare regimens.

66   *Pediatric Nursing: Scope and Standards of Practice*

Appendix B. Pediatric Nursing: Scope and Standards of Practice (2008)

- Makes decisions and initiates actions on behalf of children and their families in an ethical manner, taking into consideration the values of the child and family.
- Ensures informed consent or age-appropriate assent for procedures, treatment, and research, as appropriate.
- Serves as an advocate for the child and family in developing policies and in providing care to the child and family.
- Contributes to the creation of individual and system responses to resolution of ethical dilemmas.
- Advocates for a process of ongoing ethical inquiry into patient care practices where varying perspectives are acknowledged and validated.

Appendix B. Pediatric Nursing: Scope and Standards of Practice (2008)

The content in this appendix is not current and is of historical significance only.

STANDARD 13. RESEARCH, EVIDENCE-BASED PRACTICE, AND CLINICAL SCHOLARSHIP

The pediatric nurse integrates research findings into practice and, where appropriate, participates in the generation of new knowledge.

Measurement Criteria:

The Pediatric Nurse:

- Utilizes the best available evidence, including research findings, to guide practice decisions.

- Protects the rights of all children and families involved in research studies.

- Actively participates in research activities at various levels appropriate to the nurse's level of education, position, and practice environment. Such activities may include:

    - Identifying clinical problems or questions suitable for nursing research.

    - Identifying possible candidates to be enrolled in studies.

    - Participating in data collection.

    - Participating in a formal committee or program.

    - Sharing research activities and findings with peers and others.

    - Conducting research.

    - Critically analyzing and interpreting research for application to practice.

    - Translating research findings in the development of policies, procedures, and standards of practice for the delivery of pediatric health care.

    - Incorporating research as a basis for learning.

Appendix B. Pediatric Nursing: Scope and Standards of Practice (2008)

Additional Measurement Criteria for the Advanced Practice Pediatric Nurse:

The Advanced Practice Pediatric Nurse:

- Contributes to nursing knowledge by conducting or synthesizing research that discovers, examines, and evaluates knowledge, theories, criteria, and creative approaches to improve healthcare practice.

- Formally and informally disseminates research findings through practice, education, presentations, publications, consultation, and journal clubs.

The content in this appendix is not current and is of historical significance only.

Appendix B. *Pediatric Nursing: Scope and Standards of Practice (2008)*

Standards of Pediatric Nursing Practice

69

STANDARD 14. RESOURCE UTILIZATION

The pediatric nurse considers factors related to safety, effectiveness, cost, and impact on practice in planning and delivering patient care.

Measurement Criteria:

The Pediatric Nurse:

- Evaluates factors such as safety, effectiveness, availability, cost and benefits, efficiencies, and impact on practice when choosing practice options that would result in the same expected outcome.

- Assists the child and family in identifying and securing appropriate and available services to address health-related needs.

- Assigns or delegates tasks, based on the needs and condition of the child, potential for harm, stability of the child's condition, complexity of the task, and predictability of the outcome.

- Assists the child and family in becoming informed consumers about the options, costs, risks, and benefits of treatment and care.

- Assists the family in identifying and accessing resources for pediatric patients requiring long-term or rehabilitative care.

Additional Measurement Criteria for the Advanced Practice Pediatric Nurse:

The Advanced Practice Pediatric Nurse:

- Utilizes organizational and community resources to formulate multidisciplinary or interdisciplinary plans of care.

- Develops innovative solutions for child healthcare problems that address effective resource utilization and maintenance of quality.

- Develops evaluation strategies to demonstrate cost effectiveness, cost–benefit, and efficiency factors associated with pediatric nursing practice.

- Develops evaluation methods to measure safety and effectiveness for interventions and outcomes.

- Promotes activities that assist others, as appropriate, in becoming informed about costs, risks, and benefits of care or of the plan of care and solution.

70   *Pediatric Nursing: Scope and Standards of Practice*

Appendix B. Pediatric Nursing: Scope and Standards of Practice (2008)

- Initiates ongoing activities to analyze patient care systems in an effort to improve the quality of care provided to children and their families.

- Uses aggregate data, in cooperation with others, to develop or revise systems to avoid duplication of or gaps in service.

- Advocates for the removal of barriers to care and for optimal care for the child and family.

- Develops innovative solutions and applies strategies to obtain appropriate resources for nursing initiatives.

- Secures organizational resources to ensure a work environment conducive to completing the identified plan of care and outcomes.

Standards of Pediatric Nursing Practice 71

STANDARD 15. LEADERSHIP

The pediatric nurse provides leadership in the professional practice setting and the profession.

Measurement Criteria:

The Pediatric Nurse:

- Engages in teamwork as a team leader or team member.

- Works to create and maintain healthy work environments in local, regional, national, or international communities.

- Displays the ability to define a clear vision, the associated goals, and a plan of care to implement and measure progress.

- Demonstrates a commitment to continuous, lifelong learning for self and others.

- Teaches others to succeed by mentoring and other strategies.

- Exhibits creativity and flexibility through times of change.

- Demonstrates energy, excitement, and a passion for quality work.

- Willingly accepts and is accountable for errors by self and others, thereby creating a culture in which risk-taking is not only safe, but also expected.

- Inspires loyalty through the valuing of people as the most precious asset in an organization.

- Directs the coordination of care across settings and among care-givers, including oversight of licensed and unlicensed personnel in any assigned or delegated tasks.

- Serves in key roles in the work setting by participating on committees, councils, and administrative teams.

- Promotes advancement of the profession through participation in professional organizations.

Additional Measurement Criteria for the Advanced Practice Pediatric Nurse:

The Advanced Practice Pediatric Nurse:

- Works to influence decision-making bodies to improve child health-care, health services, and policies.

- Provides direction to enhance the effectiveness of the multidisciplinary healthcare team.

- Initiates and revises protocols or guidelines to reflect evidence-based practice, accepted changes in care management, or to address emerging problems.

- Promotes communication of information and advancement of the profession through writing, publishing, and presentations for professional or lay audiences.

- Designs innovations to effect change in practice and improve health outcomes.

Standards of Pediatric Nursing Practice

73

STANDARD 16. ADVOCACY

The pediatric nurse is an advocate for the pediatric client and family.

Measurement Criteria:

The Pediatric Nurse:

- Advocates for organizational, environmental, and practice changes to ensure that the unique health needs of children are met.

- Assists children and families to adjust to the changing healthcare environment.

- Protects the human and legal rights of the pediatric patient and family.

- Serves as a leader for the purpose of influencing healthcare practice and policy in the care of children, families, and communities.

- Assists the pediatric client and family in decision-making regarding healthcare choices.

- Provides pediatric clients and families with informed choices.

- Advocates for the child, and works with families, social service agencies, and the courts when there is concern about child abuse, neglect, or other forms of family violence.

- Raises public awareness about issues related to the health care of children and families.

- Participates in legislative agendas that improve healthcare access and provision of care to children and families.

- Demonstrates an understanding of the laws that impact confidentiality in the provision of care (e.g., Health Insurance Portability Accountability Act [HIPAA] and Family Educational Rights and Privacy Act [FERPA]).

- Advocates for children and parents to assure they are afforded the rights guaranteed to them by federal law (e.g., Individuals with Disabilities Education Act [IDEA]).

Appendix B. Pediatric Nursing: Scope and Standards of Practice (2008)

Additional measurement criteria for the Advanced Practice Pediatric Nurse:

The Advanced Practice Pediatric Nurse:

- Advances the profession through enhancing public awareness and health professional familiarity with the advanced practice pediatric nursing role and scope of practice.

Standards of Pediatric Nursing Practice 75

REFERENCES

Alexander, J.E. et al. (1998). Virginia Henderson: Definition of nursing. In A. Tomey & Alligood, M. (Eds.), *Nursing theorists and their work* (4th ed., pp. 99–111). St. Louis: Mosby.

American Association of Colleges of Nursing. (1996). *The essentials of master's education for advanced practice nursing.* Washington, DC: AACN.

American Association of Colleges of Nursing. (1998). *The essentials of baccalaureate education for professional nursing practice.* Washington, DC: AACN.

American Association of Colleges of Nursing. (2006). *The essentials of doctoral education for advanced nursing practice.* Washington, DC: AACN.

American Nurses Association. (2001). *Code of ethics for nurses with interpretive statements.* Silver Spring, MD: Nursesbooks.org.

American Nurses Association. (2003). *Nursing's social policy statement* (2nd ed.). Silver Spring, MD: Nursesbooks.org.

American Nurses Association. (2004). *Nursing: Scope and standards of practice.* Silver Spring, MD: Nursesbooks.org.

American Nurses Association & Society of Pediatric Nurses. (2003). *Scope and standards of pediatric nursing practice.* Silver Spring, MD: Nursesbooks.org.

American Public Health Association, Inc. (1955). *Health supervision of young children.* New York, NY: APHA.

Association of Camp Nurses. (2005). *The scope and standards of camp nursing practice* (2nd ed.). Bernidji, MN: Association of Camp Nurses.

77

Appendix B. Pediatric Nursing: Scope and Standards of Practice (2008)

Association of Social Work Boards (ASWB), Federation of State Boards of Physical Therapy (FSBPT), Federation of State Medical Boards (FSMB), National Board for Certification in Occupational Therapy (NMCOT), National Council of State Boards of Nursing, Inc. (NCSBN), & the National Association of Boards of Pharmacy (NABP). (2007). *Changes in health-care professions' scope of practice: Legislative considerations.* Retrieved April 19, 2008, from https://www.ncsbn.org/ScopeofPractice.pdf

Betz, C. L. (2003). Nurse's role in promoting health transitions for adolescents and young adults with developmental disabilities. *Nursing Clinics of North America, 38*(2), 271–89.

Betz, C.L. (2004a). Transition of adolescents with special health care needs: Review and analysis of the literature. *Issues in Comprehensive Pediatric Nursing, 27,* 179–241.

Betz, C. L. (2004b). Adolescents in transition of adult care: Why the concern? *Nursing Clinics of North America, 39*(4), 681–713.

Brady, N. & Lewin, L. (2007). Evidence-based practice in nursing: Bridging the gap between research and practice. *Journal of Pediatric Health Care, 21,* 53–56.

Breuner, C.C., Barry, P.J., & Kemper, K.J. (1998). Alternative medicine by homeless youth. *Archives Pediatric Adolescent Medicine, 152,* 1071–1075.

Caplan, G. (1961). *An approach to community mental health.* New York, NY: Grune and Stratton.

Children's Defense Fund. (2006). *Improving children's health: Understanding children's health disparities and promising approaches to address them.* Washington, DC: CDF.

Connolly, C. (2005). Growth and development of a specialty: The professionalization of child health care. *Pediatric Nursing, 31,* 211–215.

Consensus Panel on Genetic/Genomic Nursing Competencies. (2006). *Essential nursing competencies and curricula guidelines for genetics and genomics.* Silver Spring, MD: American Nurses Association.

The content in this appendix is not current and is of historical significance only.

78   ***Pediatric Nursing: Scope and Standards of Practice***

Cowell, J. & Swartwout, K. (2006). Healthcare home: Ensuring access to a regular healthcare provider. In M. Craft-Rosenberg and M. Krajicek (Eds.), *Nursing excellence for children and families* (pp. 23–40). New York, NY: Springer Publishing Co.

Craft-Rosenberg, M. & Krajicek, M. (2006). *Nursing excellence for children and families.* New York, NY: Springer Publishing Co.

Crowley, A. (2001). Child care health consultation: An ecological model. *Journal of the Society of Pediatric Nurses, 6* (4), 170–181.

Deatrick, J. (2006). Family partnerships in nursing care. In M. Craft-Rosenberg and Krajicek, M. (Eds.), *Nursing excellence for children and families* (pp. 41–56). New York, NY: Springer Publishing Co.

Deatrick, J. & Knafl, K. (1990). Management behaviors: Day-to-day adjustments to childhood chronic conditions. *Journal of Pediatric Nursing, 5,* 15–22.

Duderstadt, K., Hughes, K., Soobader, M., & Newacheck, P. (2006). The impact of public insurance expansions on children's access and use of care. *Pediatrics, 118* (4), 1676–1682.

Field, M.J. & Behrman, R.E. (Eds.), (2003). *When children die: Improving palliative and end-of-life are for children and their families.* Institute of Medicine of the National Academies. Washington, DC: National Academies Press.

Gance-Cleveland, B. (2001). Pediatric nurses: Advocates against youth violence. *Journal of the Society of Pediatric Nurses, 6* (3), 133–142.

Gance-Cleveland, B., Costin, D.K. & Degenstein, J.A. (2003). School-based health centers: Statewide quality improvement program. *Journal of Nursing Care Quality, 18*(4), 288–94.

Guilday, P. (2000). School nursing practice today: Implications for the future. *Journal of School Nursing, 16*(5), 25–31.

Harrison, T.W. (2003). Adolescent homosexuality and concerns regarding disclosure. *Journal of School Health, 73* (3), 107–112.

Pediatric Nursing: Scope of Practice 79

Henderson, V. (1964). The nature of nursing. *American Journal of Nursing, 64*(8), 62–68.

Institute of Medicine. (2001). *Crossing the quality chasm: A new health system for the 21st century*. Washington, DC: National Academy of Sciences.

Knafl, K., Breitmayer, B., Gallo, A., & Zoeller, L. (1996). Family response to childhood chronic illness: Description of management styles. *Journal of Pediatric Nursing, 11*, 315–326.

Knafl, K. & Deatrick, J. (2002). The challenge of normalization for families of children with chronic conditions. *Pediatric Nursing, 28*, 48–56.

Lewandowski, L. & Tesler, M. (2003). *Family-centered care: Putting it into action – the SPN/ANA guide to family-centered care*. Washington, DC: Nursesbooks.org.

Melynk, B. & Fineout-Overholt, E. (Ed.), (2005). *Evidence-based practice in nursing and health care*. Philadelphia, PA: Lippincott, Williams and Wilkins.

Melnyk, B. & Moldenhauer, Z. (2006). *The KySSSM guide to child and adolescent mental health screening, early intervention and health promotion*. Cherry Hill, NJ: National Association of Pediatric Nurse Practitioners.

Miles, M.S. (1996). News from the society: A historical perspective. *Journal of the Society of Pediatric Nurses, 1*(1), 46–47.

Murphy, M. (1990). A brief history of pediatric nurse practitioners and NAPNAP: 1964–1990. *Journal of Pediatric Health Care, 4*, 332–338.

National Association of Children's Hospitals and Related Institutions. (2006). *All children need children's hospitals*. Retrieved April 19, 2008, from http://www.childrenshospitals.net/AM/Template.cfm?Section= Fact_Sheet&Template=/TaggedPage/TaggedPageDisplay.cfm&TPLID= 61&ContentID=2262.

Appendix B. Pediatric Nursing: Scope and Standards of Practice (2008)

National Association of Clinical Nurse Specialists. (2004). *Statement on clinical nurse specialist practice and education*. (2nd ed.). Harrisburg, PA: NACNS.

National Association of Neonatal Nurses. (2006). *Education standards for neonatal nurse practitioner programs*. Glenview, IL: NANN. Retrieved May 29, 2008, from http://www.nann.org/pdf/NNP_Standards.pdf National Association of Pediatric Nurse Practitioners. (2002a). NAPNAP position statement on age parameters for PNP practice. *Journal of Pediatric Health Care, 16*, A36.

National Association of Pediatric Nurse Practitioners. (2002b). NAPNAP position statement on the pediatric health care home. *Journal of Pediatric Health Care, 17*, A22.

National Association of Pediatric Nurse Practitioners. (2004a). NAPNAP position statement on protection of children involved in research studies. *Journal of Pediatric Health Care, 18*, A20–A21.

National Association of Pediatric Nurse Practitioners. (2004b). *Scope and standards of practice: Pediatric nurse practitioner (PNP)*. Cherry Hill, NJ: NAPNAP.

National Association of Pediatric Nurse Practitioners. (2005a). NAPNAP position statement on the acute care nurse practitioner. *Journal of Pediatric Health Care, 19*, A38–A39.

National Association of Pediatric Nurse Practitioners. (2005b). NAPNAP position statement on school-based and school-linked centers. *Journal of Pediatric Health Care, 19*, A25–A26

National Association of Pediatric Nurse Practitioners. (2006a). NAPNAP position statement on health risks and needs of gay, lesbian, bisexual, transgender and questioning (GLBTQ) adolescents. *Journal of Pediatric Health Care, 20*, A29–A30.

National Association of Pediatric Nurse Practitioners. (2006b). *Healthy Eating and Activity Together (HEAT™) clinical practice guideline: Identifying and preventing overweight in childhood*. Cherry Hill, NJ: NAPNP.

Pediatric Nursing: Scope of Practice   81

Appendix B. Pediatric Nursing: Scope and Standards of Practice (2008)

National Association of Pediatric Nurse Practitioners. (2007). NAPNAP position statement on access to care. *Journal of Pediatric Health Care, 21*, A35–A36.

National Association of School Nurses. (2002). *Position statement: Education, licensure, and certification of school nurses.* Retrieved April 19, 2008, from http://www.nasn.org/Portals/0/positions/2002pseducation.pdf

National Association of School Nurses. (2003). *Access to a school nurse.* Retrieved May 29, 2008, from http://www.nasn.org/Portals/0/statements/resolutionaccess.pdf

National Association of School Nurses. (2006). *School nursing management of students with chronic health conditions.* Scarborough, ME: NASN. Retrieved June 27, 2007, from: http://www.nasn.org/Default.aspx?tabid=351

National Association of School Nurses & American Nurses Association. (2005). *School nursing: Scope and standards of practice.* Silver Spring, MD: Nursesbooks.org.

National Center for Complementary and Alternative Medicine (NCCAM). (2007). *CAM basics.* Retrieved April 19, 2008, from http://nccam.nih.gov/health/whatiscam/.

National Organization of Nurse Practitioner Faculties. (2006a). *Domains and core competencies of nurse practitioner practice.* Washington, DC: NONPF.

National Organization of Nurse Practitioner Faculties. (2006b). *Advanced nursing practice: Curriculum guidelines and program standards for nurse practitioner education.* Washington, DC: NONPF.

National Panel for Acute Care Nurse Practitioner Competencies. (2004). *Acute care nurse practitioner competencies.* Washington, DC: NONPF.

Nehring, W. M., Roth, S. P., Natvig, D., Betz, C. L., Savage, T., & Krajicek, M. (2004). *Intellectual and developmental disabilities nursing: Scope and standards of practice.* American Nurses Association and the American Association on Mental Retardation. Washington, DC: Nursesbooks.org.

Nelson, J. (2003). Providing health care to lesbian, gay, bisexual and transgender adolescents. In D.A. Gaffney & C. Roye (Eds.), *Adolescent Sexual Development and Sexuality.* Kingston, NJ: Civic Research Institute, Inc.

Ottolini, M., Hamburger, E., Loprieto, J., Coleman, R.H., Sachs, H.C., Madden, R., & Brasseux, C. (1999, May). *Alternative medicine use among children in the Washington, DC, area.* Paper presented at the meeting of the Pediatric Academic Societies. San Francisco, CA.

Pearson, L. (2007). The Pearson Report: A national overview of nurse practitioner legislation and healthcare issues. *American Journal for Nurse Practitioners, 11*(2), 10–101.

Percy, M. & Sperhac, A. (2007). State regulations for the pediatric nurse practitioner in acute care. *Journal of Pediatric Health Care, 21* (1), 29–43.

Plotnick, J. (2007, March). *Responding globally to the world's children: Addressing health care needs.* Symposium conducted at the annual meeting of the National Association of Pediatric Nurse Practitioners. Lake Buena Vista, FL.

Pridham, K. F. (1993). Anticipatory guidance of parents of new infants: Potential contribution of the internal working model construct. *Image: Journal of Nursing Scholarship, 25,* 49–56.

Ramler, M., Nakatsukasa-Ono., W., Loe, C. & Harris, K. (2006). *The influence of child care health consultants in promoting children's health and well-being: A report on selected resources.* Retrieved April 19, 2008, from http://hcccnsc.edc.org/resources/data/CC_lit_review_Screen_All.pdf

Sackett, D.L., Straus, S.E., Richardson, W.S., Rosenberg, W., & Haynes, R. B. (2000). *Evidence-based medicine: How to practice and teach EBM.* Edinburgh, UK: Churchill Livingstone.

Appendix B. Pediatric Nursing: Scope and Standards of Practice (2008)

Safriet, B.J. (1992). Health care dollars and regulatory sense: The role of advanced practice nursing. *Yale Journal on Regulation, 9*(2), 417–488.

Safriet, B.J. (2002). Closing the gap between *can* and *may* in health-care providers' scopes of practice: A primer for policymakers. *Yale Journal on Regulation, 19*: 301–334.

Shelton, T. L. & Sepanek, J. S. (1994). *Family-centered care for children needing specialized health and developmental services.* Bethesda, MD: Association for the Care of Children's Health.

Society of Pediatric Nurses. (2004). *The role of the staff nurse in protecting children and families involved in research.* Retrieved April 19, 2008, from https://www.pedsnurses.org/index.php?option=com_docman&task=doc_view&gid=68&Itemid=117.

Sullivan, E.J. (2004). *Becoming influential: A guide for nurses.* Upper Saddle River, NJ: Pearson Education, Inc.

Taylor, M. (2006). Mapping the literature of pediatric nursing. *Journal of the Medical Library Association 94* (Suppl. 2), E-128–E-136.

U.S. Department of Health and Human Services. (2002). *Children's health highlights.* (AHRQ Publication No. 02-P005).

U.S. Department of Health and Human Services. (2005). *Selected findings on child and adolescent health care hrom the 2004 National Healthcare Quality/Disparities Reports.* (AHRQ Publication No. 05-P011).

Woodring, B. C. & Pridham, K.F. (Ed.), (1998). *Standards and guidelines for pre-licensure and early professional education for the nursing care of children and their families. (Revised).* Department of Health and Human Services, Bureau of Maternal and Child Health, Document #H112R77. Washington, DC: U.S. Government Printing Office.

World Health Organization. (2007). *International classification of functioning, disability and health—Children and youth version (ICF–CY).* Geneva: WHO.

Appendix B. Pediatric Nursing: Scope and Standards of Practice (2008)

The content in this appendix is not current and is of historical significance only.

Index

A

accountability in pediatric nursing practice (ethical provision), 40

adolescence to adulthood passage, 23–24

advanced practice registered nurses (APRNs)
  accountability of, 7–8
  competencies, 47, 48, 49, 51–52, 54, 55–56, 57–58, 61–62, 65–66, 67, 70–71, 73, 74–75, 77, 78–79, 80, 82
  definition of, 19
  education, 32–33, 34
  pediatric nursing practice and, 19–21
  regulation of, 35
  regulatory challenges for, 21–22
  roles of, 35

advancement of the profession in pediatric nursing practice, 41–42

advocacy, 7–8. *See also* advocacy in pediatric nursing practice
  competencies, 81–82
  in health care, 34
  school nurses, 39
  Standards of Professional Performance, 7–8, 81–82
  student nurses, 28
  tool kits, 43

advocacy [2008], 177–178

advocacy in pediatric care [2008], 140–141

advocacy in pediatric nursing practice, 7, 13, 17, 41, 43–44

competencies involved in, 53, 55, 58, 64, 71, 79, 80
  ethical provision on, 39–40
  by state and national organizations, 43

Air and Surface Transport Nurses Association (ASTNA), 30

ambulatory care settings, 27–28

American Association of Colleges of Nursing (AACN)
  on future of APRN and CNS education, 33–34
  The Essentials of Baccalaureate Education for Professional Nursing Practice, 32
  The Essentials of Doctoral Education for Advanced Nursing Practice, 34
  The Essentials of Master's Education for Advanced Practice Nursing, 32–33

American Nurses Association (ANA), xi, xiii, 83, 84, 85, 86, 87, 88
  Code of Ethics for Nurses with Interpretive Statements, 37–38
  on regulation of nursing practice, 35
  on single scope of nursing practice, 35

American Nurses Credentialing Center (ANCC), 18, 20, 36
  pediatric nursing certification and, 18

American Pediatric Surgical Nurses Association (APSNA), xi, 26

assessment
  competencies, 45–47
  criteria for, 89–91
  Standards of Practice, 45–47

assessment [2008], 143–146

Association of Faculties of Pediatric
Nurse Practitioners (AFPNP), xi, 21
Association of Pediatric Gastroenterology
and Nutrition Nurses (APGNN), xi
ASTNA (Air and Surface Transport
Nurses Association), 30

C

CAM (complementary and alternative
medicine), 31–32
camp settings, 30
care
family-centered, 2
care coordination in pediatric nursing
practice, 7. *See also* coordination
of care
care quality. *See* quality of care in
pediatric nursing practice
care transition in pediatric nursing
practice, 23
caring for a diverse population [2008],
131
certification [2008], 136–137
certification in pediatric nursing practice,
18, 34–35, 36
certified nurse midwife (CNM), 35
certified nurse practitioner (CNP), 35
certified registered nurse anesthetist
(CRNA), 35
*Changes in Healthcare Professions'
Scope of Practice: Legislative
Considerations,* xi–xii
clinical nurse specialists (CNS), 35
core competencies, 33
clinical nurse specialists in pediatric
nursing (PCNS), 19–20
*Code of Ethics for Nurses with Interpretive
Statements* (ANA), 37–38
collaboration. *See also* interprofessional
practice
competencies, 74–75
in patient- and family-centered care,
16
in pediatric nursing care, 16
in pediatric nursing practice (ethical
provision), 42
and school nurses, 39

Standards of Professional Performance,
74–75
collaboration in pediatric nursing
practice, 4, 7, 13, 16, 21, 24, 27,
28, 32, 42, 47, 53, 54, 58, 61, 79
collaborative practice model, 20
collegiality [2008], 167
commitment in pediatric nursing practice
to the patient (ethical provision),
38–39
to the profession, 44
communication
competencies, 70–71
Standards of Professional Performance,
70–71
communication in pediatric nursing
practice, 7, 18, 28, 42, 53, 54, 55,
57, 59, 64, 75, 80
in adolescence to adulthood passage,
23, 24
community health in pediatric nursing
practice, 1, 14, 25, 43, 53, 54, 55,
56, 72, 73, 74, 78, 80, 81
advocacy activities, 43
moral community concept, 37
settings, 28, 28–30
competencies
advanced practice registered nurses,
47, 48, 49, 51–52, 54, 55–56,
57–58, 61–62, 64, 65–66, 67,
70–71, 73, 74–75, 77, 78–79,
80, 82
advocacy, 81–82
assessment, 45–47
CNS core, 33
collaboration, 74–75
communication, 70–71
consultation, 59
coordination of care, 55–56
diagnosis, 48
education, 65–66
environmental health, 80
ethics, 63–64
evaluation, 61–62
evidence-based practice and research,
66–67
health teaching and health promotion,
57–58

implementation, 53–54
leadership, 72–73
outcomes identification, 49
planning, 50–51
prescriptive authority and treatment, 60
professional practice evaluation, 76–77
quality of practice, 68–69
resource utilization, 78–79
competencies for pediatric nursing practice, 8
complementary and alternative medicine (CAM), 31–32
complementary therapies [2008], 132–133
Consensus Model for APRN Regulation: Licensure, Accreditation, Certification and Education, xiii, 35
consultation in pediatric nursing practice, 29–30, 65, 67, 71, 74
competencies, 59
Standards of Practice, 59
consulting [2008], 157
continued commitment to the profession [2008], 141–142
continuity of care in pediatric nursing practice, 7
coordination of care
competencies, 55–56
Standards of Practice, 55–56
coordination of care and case management [2008], 154
cost-effectiveness in pediatric nursing practice, 2, 20–21, 21, 53, 56, 82
cultural issues and pediatric nursing practice, 18
cultural sensitivity in pediatric nursing practice, 4, 5, 7, 16, 22, 32, 37

D

data and data collection in pediatric nursing practice, 45, 46, 48, 51, 53, 55, 59, 61, 66, 68, 76, 79
definition and function of standards [2008], 106
development of standards [2008], 106

diagnosis
competencies, 48
Standards of Practice, 48
diagnosis [2008], 147
diagnosis in pediatric nursing practice, 47, 48, 49, 50, 51, 53, 60, 61, 69
differentiated areas of pediatric nursing practice [2008], 18–20, 121–125
dignity
in patient- and family-centered care, 16
disparities in pediatric nursing practice, 12–13
health homes and, 13
diverse populations in pediatric nursing practice, 12–13, 18, 22
Doctor of Nursing Practice (DNP), 34
documentation in pediatric nursing practice, 48, 49, 51, 52, 53, 54, 55, 61, 68, 74, 75
duties to self and others in pediatric nursing practice
ethical provision, 40–41

E

education
competencies, 65–66
Standards of Professional Performance, 65–66
education [2008], 133–136, 166
education in nursing practice
APRNs, 34
doctoral preparation for, 34
Doctor of Nursing Practice (DNP), 34
genetics and genomics in, 32
education in pediatric nursing practice, 32–35
education of patients in pediatric nursing practice, 7
environmental health
competencies, 80
Standards of Professional Performance, 80
Essential Nursing Competencies and Curricula Guidelines for Genetics and Genomics (Consensus Panel on Genetic/Genomic Competencies), 32

The Essentials of Baccalaureate Education
for Professional Nursing Practice
(AACN), 32
The Essentials of Doctoral Education for
Advanced Nursing Practice (AACN),
34
The Essentials of Master's Education for
Advanced Practice Nursing (AACN),
32–33
ethical issues in pediatric care [2008],
139–140, 169–170
ethics. See also Code of Ethics for Nurses
with Interpretive Statements
competencies, 63–64
Standards of Professional Performance,
63–64
ethics in pediatric nursing practice, 7, 18,
37–44
advancement of the profession, 41–42
advocacy for the patient, 39–40
code of ethics and, 37–38
collaboration, 42
commitment to the patient, 38–39
duties to self and others, 40–41
ethical environment of work setting,
41
moral community concept, 37
promotion of the nursing profession,
43
respect for the individual, 38
responsibility and accountability for
practice, 40
social justice, 43
evaluation
competencies, 61–62
Standards of Practice, 61–62
evaluation [2008], 160–161
evidence-based care and research in
pediatric nursing practice, 7, 8, 17,
19, 41
evidence-based practice [2008],
118–120
evidence-based practice and research
in pediatric nursing practice, 7,
16–17
competencies, 66–67 ·
Standards of Professional Performance,
66–67

F

families in pediatric nursing practice, 18
advocating for, 13
family
definition of, 15
family-centered care and, 15
family-centered care, 2, 15. See
also patient- and family-centered
care
key elements of, 17
financial issues in pediatric nursing
practice, 21
function of the scope of practice
statement [2008], 106
The Future of Nursing: Leading Change,
Advancing Health (IOM report), xii,
22

G

gay, lesbian, bisexual, transgender,
or questioning their sexual
orientation/gender identity
(GLBTQ) youth, 22–23
genetics and genomics in nursing
education, 32
GLBTQ (gay, lesbian, bisexual,
transgender, or questioning their
sexual orientation/gender identity)
youth, 22–23
global perspectives of pediatric nursing
[2008], 132
global perspectives of pediatric nursing
practice, 31
guidelines in pediatric nursing practice,
8, 111
for education, 32
quality and outcome for children and
families, 13, 14

H

health and safety
promotion of, 40–41
health and safety of the patient. See
also safety
ethical provision, 39–40

healthcare homes, 13–14
  implementation of, 15
healthcare transitions in pediatric nursing
    practice, xiii, 23–24
health teaching and health promotion
    competencies, 57–58
  Standards of Practice, 57–58
health teaching and health promotion,
    restoration and maintenance
    [2008], 155–156
hospice and palliative care settings,
    26–27

I

implementation
  competencies, 53–54
  Standards of Practice, 53–54
implementation [2008], 152–153
information sharing
  in patient- and family-centered care,
    16
inpatient and acute care settings for
    pediatric nursing practice, 25
International Classification of
    Functioning, Disability, and
    Health–Children and Youth Version
    (ICF–CY), 5

L

leadership
  competencies, 72–73
  Standards of Professional Performance,
    72–73
leadership [2008], 175–176
leadership in pediatric nursing practice,
    8, 16
legal issues in pediatric nursing practice,
    21, 60, 63, 81
licensure for registered nurses, 35

M

measurement criteria [2008], 111
mental health services in pediatric
    nursing practice, xiii, 1, 2
  community, 14
  healthcare homes and, 13

school nursing and, 29
minorities and the poor in pediatric
    nursing practice, 12–13
moral community concept in pediatric
    nursing practice, 37

N

National Association of Clinical Nurse
    Specialists (NACNS), 19–20
  pediatric nursing and, 19–20
  *Statement on CNS Practice and
    Education,* 33
National Association of Neonatal Nurses
    (NANN), xiii, 86
National Association of Pediatric Nurse
    Practitioners (NAPNAP), xi, 86–88
National Health Interview Survey
    (2007), 31–32
  complementary and alternative (CAM)
    therapies and, 31–32
*Neonatal Nursing: Scope and Standards of
    Practice,* xiii
Nurse Practice Act, 21
nursing process and Standards of
    Practice, 6–7
nursing scope of practice, 3

O

outcomes identification
  competencies, 49
  Standards of Practice, 49
outcomes identification [2003], 148–
    149

P

participation
  in patient- and family-centered care,
    16
patient- and family-centered care, 1, 7,
    15–16
  collaboration in, 16
  development of, 2
  dignity in, 16
  information sharing in, 16
  participation in, 16
  respect in, 16

T

transport settings, 30

W

wellness in pediatric nursing practice, 23

in school settings, 29
work settings in pediatric nursing
practice, 24–31
[2008], 126–131
ethical environment, 41